Qi!

Chinese Secrets of Health, Beauty & Vitality

licence

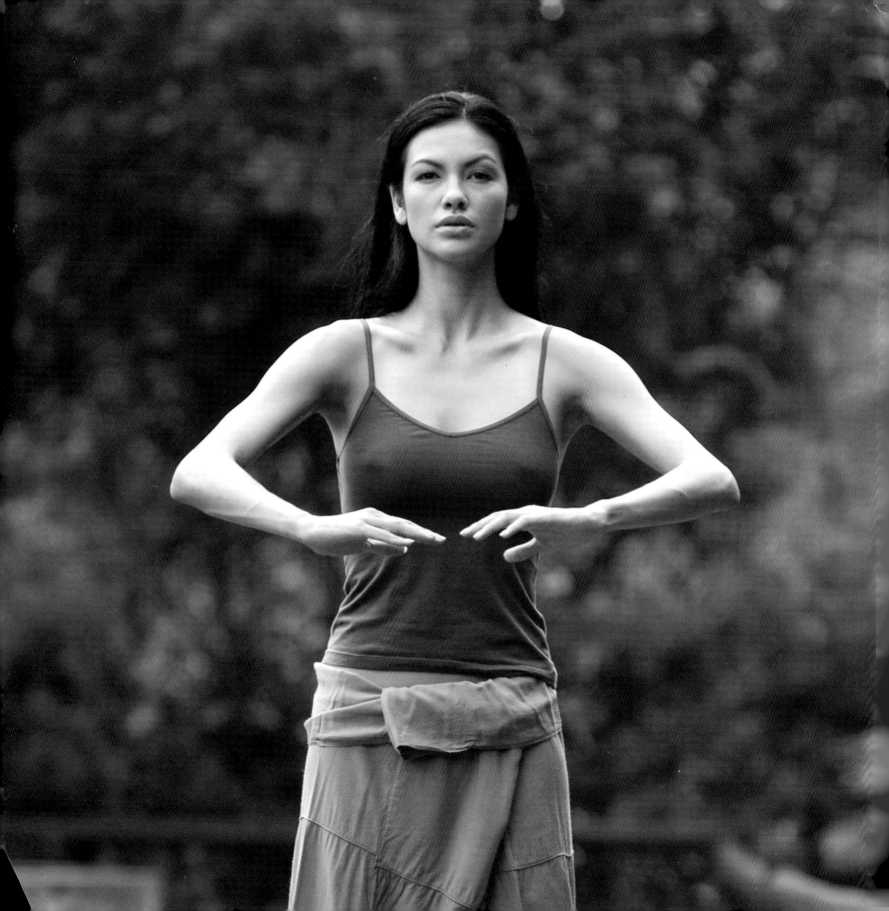

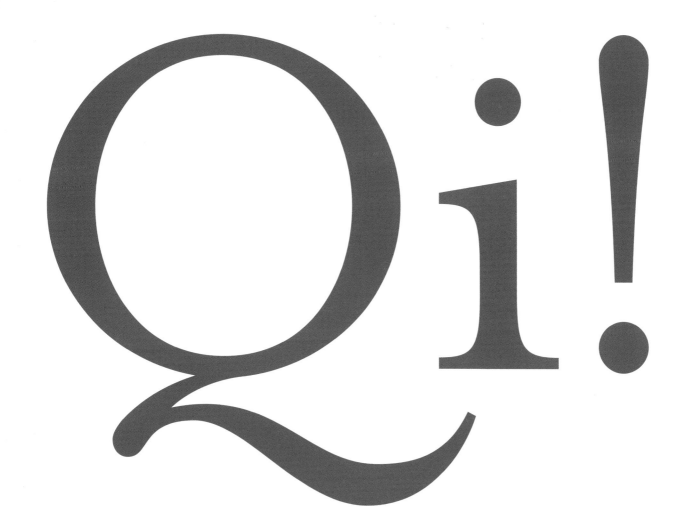

Qi!

Chinese Secrets of Health, Beauty & Vitality

By Kate O'Brien with Troy Sing, O.M.D.
Photography by Chester Ong

Qi! Chinese Secrets of Health, Beauty & Vitality

Published by C Licence Pte Ltd

Copyright © 2005 C Licence Pte Ltd

ISBN: 981-05-2923-6

Publisher/Editor: Jane Marsden

Authors: Kate O'Brien with Troy Sing, O.M.D.

Designers: Loretta Reilly, Leah Lococo and Ng Boon Hang

C Licence Pte Ltd

113 Holland Road

Singapore 278556

Tel: (65) 6474 4436

Fax: (65) 6473 8786

info@c-licence.com

Online bookstore: www.c-licence.com

Printed in Singapore by Tien Wah Press (Pte) Limited

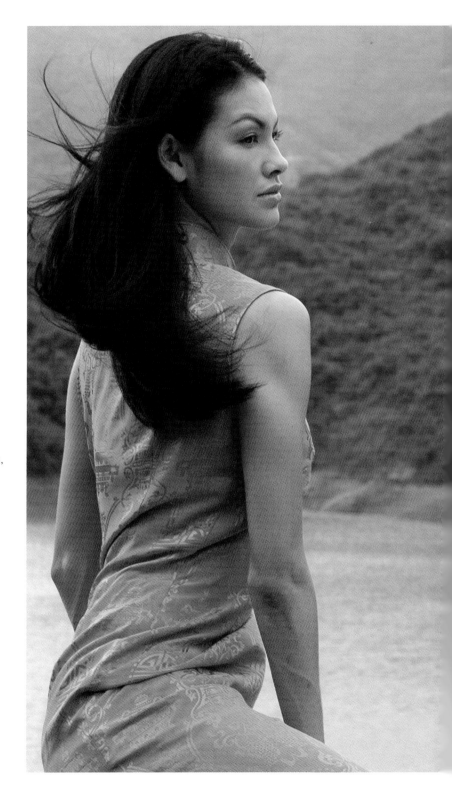

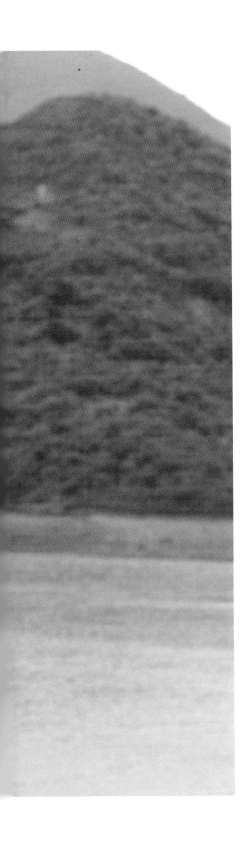

"In the universe and

achievements may

plished by starting

in life, great

easily be accom-

with small actions."

—Lao Tzu, *Tao Te Ching* (c. 1066-770BC)

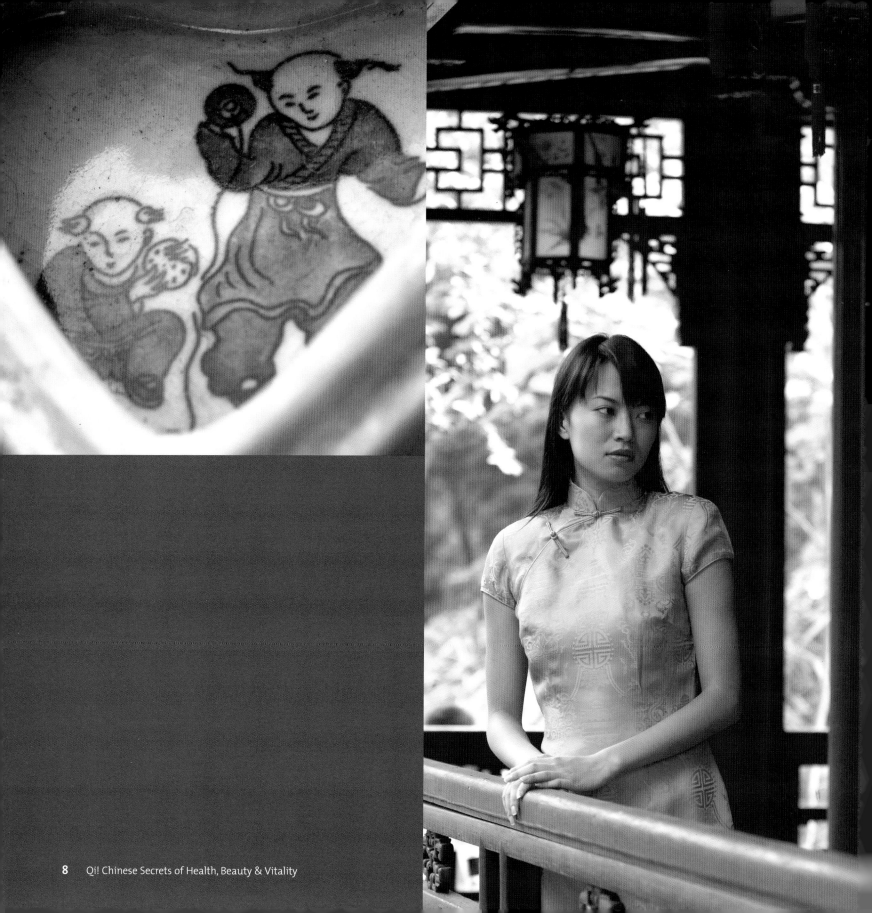

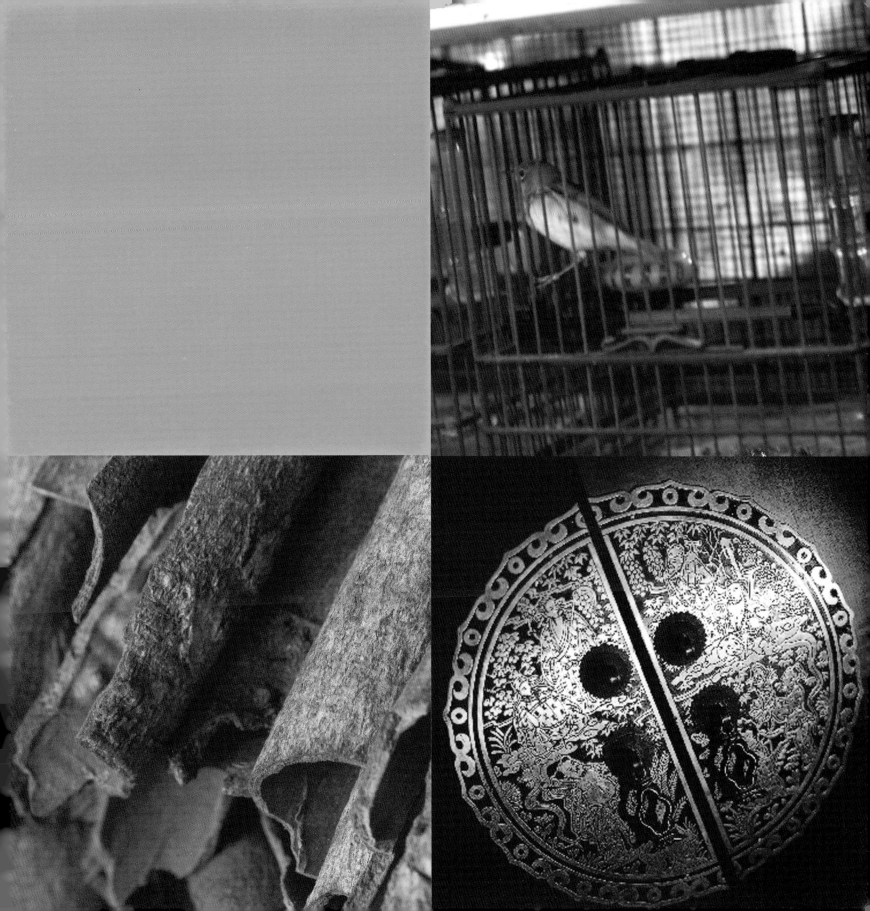

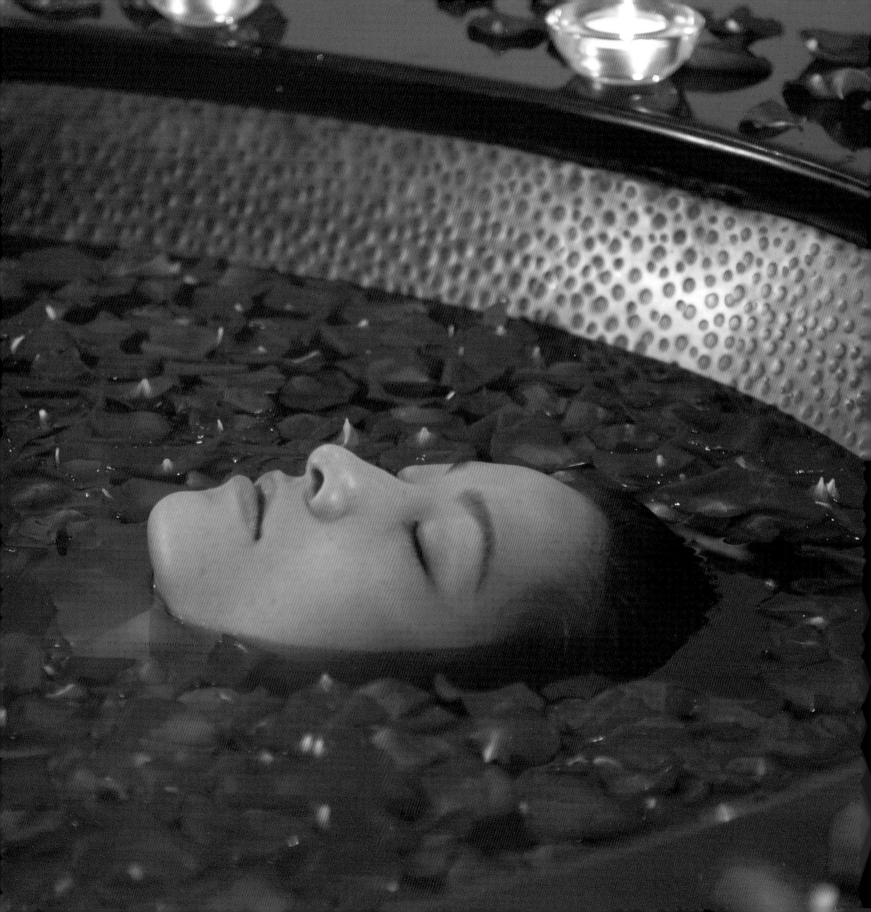

CHAPTER I

Traditional Chinese Medicine:

body, mind and spirit

"The Tao is the one
From the one comes yin and yang
From these two, creative *Qi*
From *Qi*, ten thousand things
The forms of all creation."

—Lao Tzu, *Tao Te Ching* 42, (c.1066-770BC)

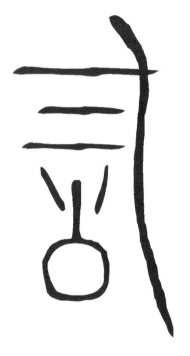

[qî]

With the present shift from Western thinking to a more integrative body-and-mind approach, Taoism, the most fundamental philosophy in the world's oldest civilization, is as relevant today as it was in classical China. While Western medicine attempts to fix a body problem by treating symptoms and disease, Chinese medicine embraces Taoism's more holistic and preventive approach focusing on diet, movement, spiritual and emotional wellbeing. It treats the body as a whole and aims to prevent illness by maintaining overall health and balance.

As the origin of Traditional Chinese Medicine (TCM) precedes the founding of Chinese culture (c. 3000BC), much misinterpretation and confusion surrounds the real meaning of yin and yang, *Qi* (also spelt how it is pronounced, i.e. *Chi*) and the Five Elements. The ideas outlined in this book are based on the 81 chapters of the *Yellow Emperor's Classic of Internal Medicine* (220BC), widely recognized by modern scholars as the authoritative manuscript of true Chinese medicine.

The Origins of Traditional Chinese Medicine

Some 5,000 years ago, the tribes of the Shang dynasty (1766-1100BC) developed a unique system for predicting seasonal change as a means of protecting their crops from the ravaging effects of the environment. These naturalists described the primal forces in terms of polar opposites or yin and yang. So began the ancient medicine of the Chinese.

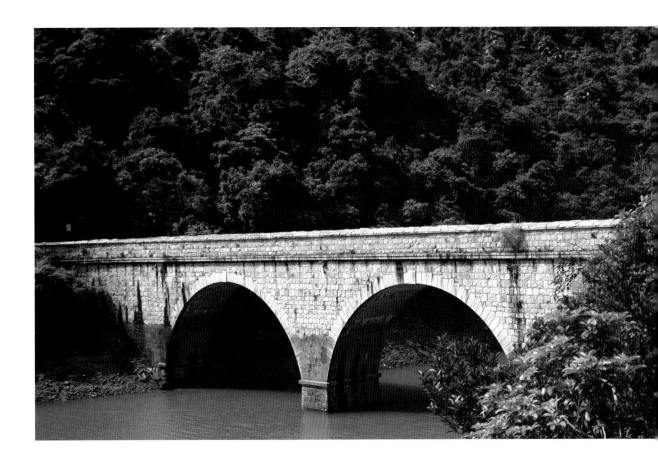

Over time the Five Elements system came into being as a method of teaching farmers when nature would be kindest to their crops. As these ancient scholars began to use the Five Elements to better understand how the human body worked in relation to the world around them, they viewed the body as a microcosm of the universe, and the fluctuations occurring within, a direct consequence of environmental change.

According to the *Yellow Emperor's Classic of Internal Medicine* (220BC), "people of ancient times understood the way of nature, the principles of yin and yang and appreciated the art of enumeration [forecasting]. They ate and drank in moderation, lived their daily lives in consistent and invariable patterns, without recklessness and without working until fatigued. Therefore they were able to maintain a healthy body and mind and, from beginning to end, live out their natural life span of at least 100 years before dying."

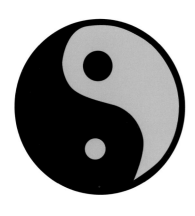

Yin and Yang

"Yin and yang are the way of heaven and earth, are fundamental to all things, are the parents of change and transformation, the origin of birth and destruction, the palace of gods and are necessarily considered in understanding the basis of health." —*Yellow Emperor's Classic of Internal Medicine* (220BC)

With the seasonal influence on the origins of Chinese medicine it is hardly surprising that yin and yang were originally depicted as the shady (yin) and sunny (yang) sides of a mountain, with yin traditionally characterized as the moon, and yang, the bright sun. Together they represent complementary poles of the same basic energy, like the positive and negative poles of an electric current.

When applied to the body, yin represents substance and yang, function. Much like a log fire whose flame is dependent on the quality and quantity of wood, our activities depend on what we eat and how we metabolize or burn this fuel. When we are young we generate more substance than we consume and we function efficiently (i.e. grow, mature and heal). However, as we get older the body's efficiency declines and we find it increasingly difficult to replenish our fuel reserves.

The classical representation of the dual nature of yin and yang, as depicted in the *taiji* symbol (top left), shows a white portion, representing yang (shown here in blue), with a smaller circle of black (yin) within, conveying the notion that one cannot exist without the other and that nothing is absolutely yin or yang but seeks a variety of interrelationships. Yin and yang nourish and foster one another; they restrain each other and they exist together.

As with everything in the natural world, both man and woman each contains aspects of yin and yang. Because of their higher body fat content and association with blood during menstruation women are perceived as more yin, while men, the primary testosterone producers with a higher percentage of muscle mass, are predominantly yang. Our bodies are in a constant state of change brought about by this yin/yang interaction. What we eat and do and the changes that take place in our daily lives have a huge effect on this relationship.

When yin and yang forces are in harmony, there is balance and optimal health—physically, emotionally and spiritually. However, if yin is dominant, illnesses related to the Chinese concepts of cold, deficiency and the interior of the body may develop. If yang is superior, conditions related to heat, excess and the exterior of the body may arise.

The Three Treasures of Chinese Medicine

In the Taoist view, the Three Treasures upon which life depends are energy *(Qi)*, essence *(Jing)* and spirit *(Shen)*. Energy is the basic life force that suffuses every cell and tissue of the body, activating its vital functions. According to Daniel Reid in *Guarding The Three Treasures* (1993), essence is the physical body of blood and flesh including its material constituents such as the essential fluids (like hormones, enzymes and neurotransmitters) and its ability to develop and reproduce. Spirit encompasses all aspects of the mind including awareness and cognition, thought and feeling, will and intent. Together these treasures function as one unit.

Qi

"Longevity is related to sufficiency of *Qi.*
If the *Qi* **is strong, life is long."**

—Wong Chong, *Essay On Balance* (400BC)

Qi, the vital breath or energy that sustains all life, has no true English-language equivalent. The Japanese refer to it as *ki*, Indian ayurvedic medicine calls it *prana* and the ancient Greeks called it *pneuma*.

Along with essence and spirit, *Qi* must be guarded and enriched through diet, lifestyle and mental health. The ancients believed that getting vital air or *Qi* to the tissues and cells through a continuously circulating blood supply was the fundamental physiological function of the body—an understanding not so far removed from present-day Western thinking. Even the most unmedically-minded know that when the heart is deprived of oxygen by a blood clot or blockage, damage occurs. However, to the Western mind, a slight aberration in blood, nutrient and oxygen circulation to the tissues or organs may not seem so significant, but to the Chinese, even the most subtle changes in flow can result in pain and disease.

When a person is in good health the movement of *Qi* and blood through the body is harmonious. However, if *Qi* and blood become blocked or slowed, the organs, tissues and cells will be deprived of the power needed to function at their best.

The Five Elements

"The five elemental energies of Wood, Fire, Earth, Metal and Water encompass all phenomena of nature. It is a symbolism that applies equally to man."

—*Yellow Emperor's Classic of Internal Medicine* (220BC)

As man is an epitome of his greater world, the human life cycle can therefore be equated with the cycles of nature with birth, growth, development, maturation and death. Often referred to as the theory of "Systematic Correspondence", the Five Elements (*wu xing*) bring together a series of seemingly unrelated objects and events, moulding them into a firm and cohesive relationship. Everything in the universe corresponds with one of the Five Elements which helps explain the effect of sounds, smells, food, the planets, seasons and emotions on our body's organs.

Based on this cohesive relationship, each element nurtures or is the "mother" of the one that follows (see page 18). Wood, for instance, is the mother of Fire. Wood burns to create fire. Wood signifies creativity and expression (e.g. the young child "creates" the adolescent, symbolized by Fire). Other elements follow suit, nurturing one another and keeping the cycle flowing harmoniously.

As a means of maintaining overall harmony and balance within the body, the "controlling cycle" was conceived to give each element the power to diminish another and prevent it from dominating: Wood (*mu*) controls Earth (*tu*), Earth controls Water (*shui*), Water controls Fire, Fire (*huo*) controls Metal (*jing*), which in turn controls Wood.

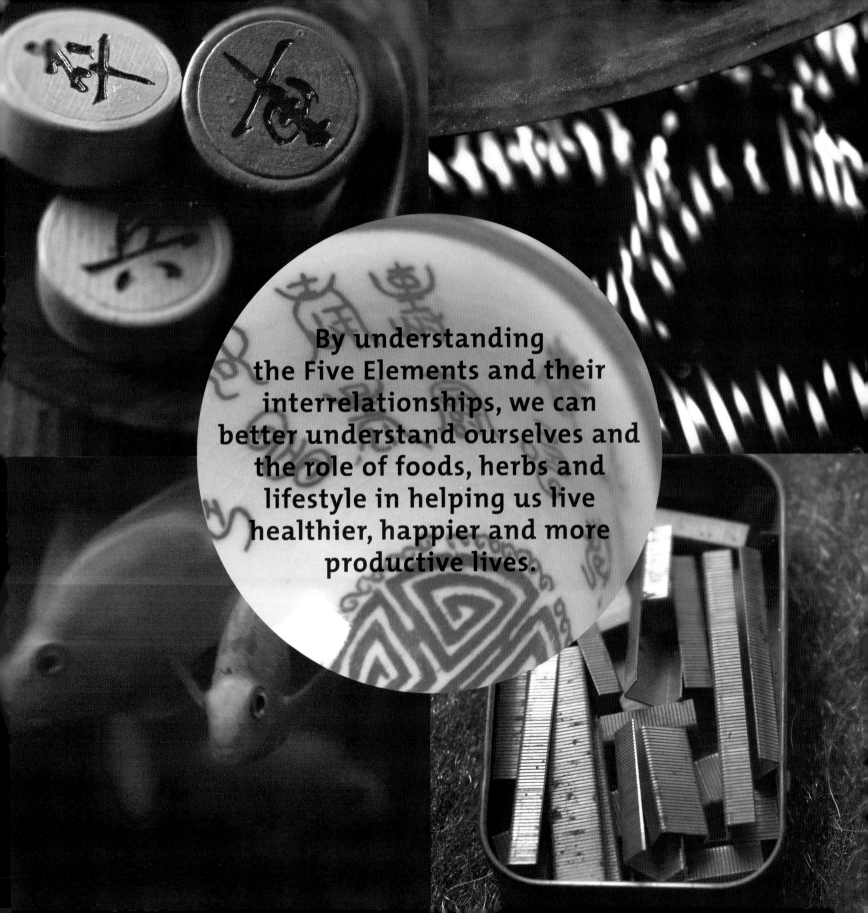

By understanding
the Five Elements and their
interrelationships, we can
better understand ourselves and
the role of foods, herbs and
lifestyle in helping us live
healthier, happier and more
productive lives.

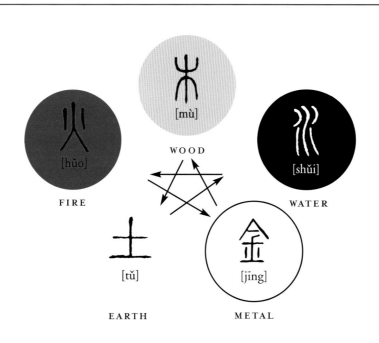

The Five Elements' Controlling Cycle

	WOOD	FIRE	EARTH	METAL	WATER
SEASON	Spring	Summer	Long Summer	Autumn	Winter
DIRECTION	East	South	Centre	West	North
DEVELOPMENT	Seed	Growth	Development	Maturation	Death
YIN ORGAN	Liver	Heart	Spleen	Lung	Kidney
YANG ORGAN	Gallbladder	Small Intestine	Stomach	Large Intestine	Bladder
EMOTION	Anger	Joy	Worry	Grief	Fear
TASTE	Sour	Bitter	Sweet	Pungent	Salty
TISSUES	Tendons	Blood	Muscles	Body hair	Bones/Marrow
SENSE ORGAN	Eyes	Tongue	Lips	Skin	Ears
COLOUR	Green	Red	Yellow	White	Black

Symbols courtesy of Banyan Tree Spa Shanghai.

Internal Organs

The ancient healers used the Five Elements and the yin and yang systems to explain how the body's internal organs (*zang fu*) function. In Chinese medicine there are two organ groups—the six bowels (yang) and the five viscera (yin), plus the pericardium (the membranous sac enclosing the heart). Yin viscera (*zang*) are solid and comprise the heart (which corresponds with the fire element), spleen (earth), lungs (metal), kidney (water) and liver (wood), while yang organs (*fu*) are hollow and include the small intestine, stomach, large intestine, bladder, gall bladder and internal membrane (a continuous membrane that separates and protects the muscles and internal organs).

Chinese medicine is an energetic rather than a mechanistic medicine and the language used describes what is happening energetically within the body. When a Chinese physician talks about the "liver" he is referring to far more than the Western concept of the liver as an "organ". He is also describing its affiliation with the wood element which inhibits earth (spleen). Thus, if the liver is not functioning well, it will affect the action of the spleen. While Western medicine refers to the symptoms (e.g. fever) of a disease, TCM groups illnesses according to the eight "syndromes" of yin-yang, exterior-interior, cold-heat and deficiency-excess, and their effect on the organs.

Living with the Seasons

"Whoever wishes to investigate medicine
should proceed thus:
In the first place, consider the seasons of the year
and what effect each of them produces."

—Hippocrates (c. 500BC)

Taoism states that there is nothing permanent except change; in Traditional Chinese Medicine, adapting to change is fundamental to continuing good health. We are at our most vulnerable when the season's energy or *Qi* changes. Day to night, weather fluctuations, changing seasons, the new moon and full moon are all important dynamics in our daily

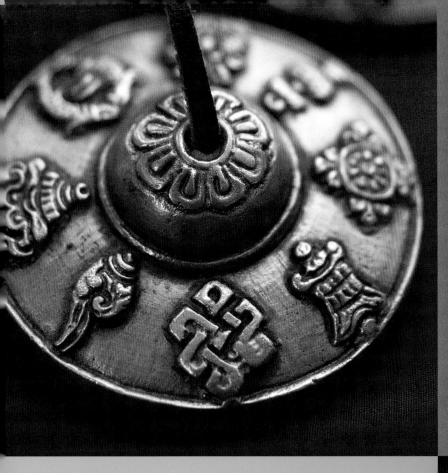

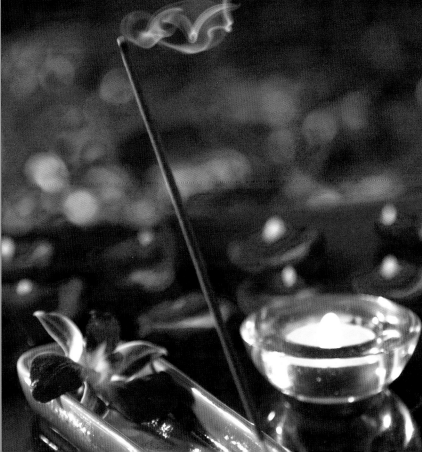

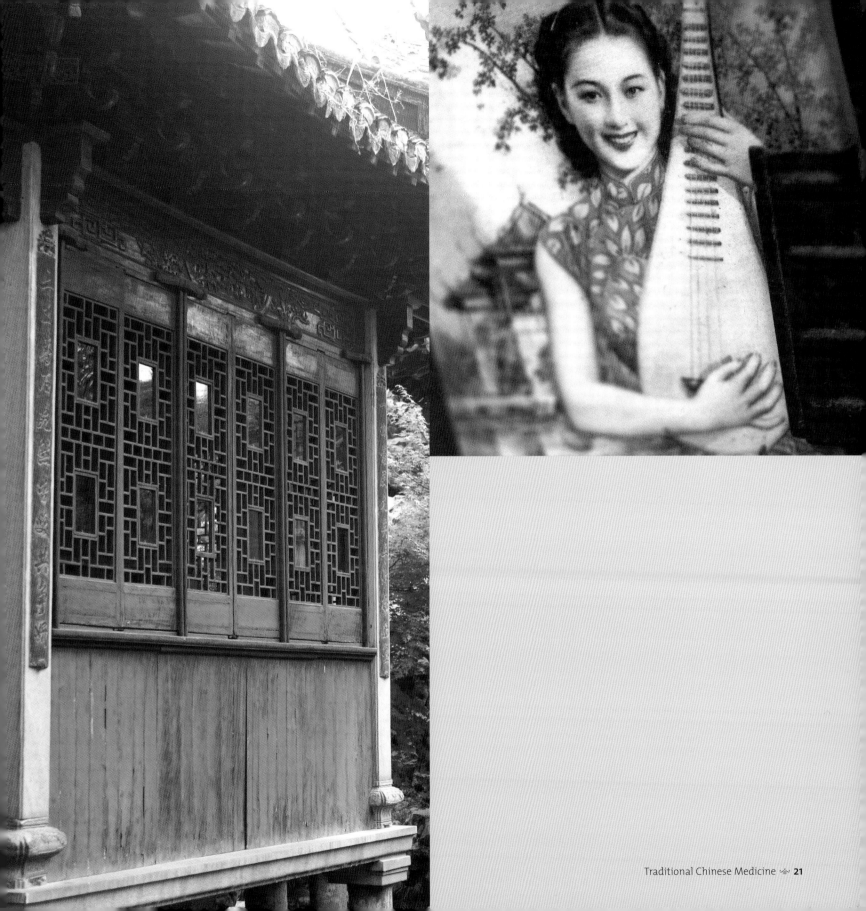

lives. These external forces also affect our internal cycles which together help regulate hormones, metabolism and menstruation and are reflected in our emotional, mental and physical wellbeing. By becoming more attuned to nature's cycles, and living and eating with the seasons, our everyday health will benefit.

While recognizing times of seasonal change as periods of greater potential stress and disease, they are also important markers for increased self-awareness and reorganization, making the body stronger and less likely to fall prey to illness.

Spring and summer are yang in nature, filled with daylight and sun. Spring is a time to revitalize the body, a time for inspiration and creativity. Alternatively, autumn and winter are yin, characterized by waning sunlight and cooler temperatures. Autumn represents ripeness and harvest while winter is a time for added warmth to protect yin.

Meridians

Qi flows along a network of 14 primary channels or meridians (*jing luo*) to empower each and every organ in the body. Twelve of these meridians (which take their names from the organs they regulate, including the stomach, heart, bladder and kidney) distribute nutrients and other biologically active essences through the body (e.g. the liver meridian services the liver organ).

Each of these meridians is made up of numerous acupoints where bundles of nerves intersect. For example, the pericardium meridian (shown opposite) follows nine points along the arm, while that of the large intestine (not shown) has 20 acupoints which trace a line through other parts of the body. Manipulation of specific acupoints through *tui na* massage, acupressure, moxibustion or acupuncture are believed to relieve disease and pain and prevent illness. For example, manipulation of the pericardium meridian's acupoint 1 (*tianchi*) near the nipple is thought to reduce chest congestion, while manipulation of the pericardium meridian's acupoint 6 (*neiguan*) just above the inner wrist is thought to regulate the heart and "clear" heat.

Exercises that manipulate the flow of *Qi* like *qi gung* and *tai chi* have been practised in a variety of forms for thousands of years. This is where movement and massage become so closely intertwined with medicine as these therapies direct the flow of *Qi* through the meridians to nourish and energize the body, keeping it in balance and health.

The Emotions in Chinese Medicine
When the key emotions of anger, joy, anxiety/worry, grief and fear are in balance, the body is stronger and healthier; intense or suppressed emotion of any kind can breed disease. Mind-body-spirit medicine excels in recognizing that certain physical ailments are deeply rooted in the emotions. This explains why, for instance, children wet their pants with fear (the emotion "fear" is associated with the kidney organ and the water element).

ANGER: The emotion of anger and the sound of shouting relate to the wood element. Expressed in a safe way it is healthy, but if suppressed can injure the liver and gall bladder leading to frustration and erratic behaviour, high blood pressure, headaches and liver complaints.

JOY: The yang heat of joy works wonders for the heart but constant stimulation results in emotional extremes from hysteria to anxiety, insomnia and intestinal upset.

Assessing Health and Preventing Disease

"To treat a disease one should determine its roots," directs the *Yellow Emperor's Classic of Internal Medicine* (220BC). Diagnosis in Chinese medicine relies on the "four examinations" of looking, listening/smelling, questioning and palpitation (pressing) of the body or measuring the pulse. Together these reveal the body's overall wellbeing which includes its emotional state, energy levels and the health of the internal organs.

In Chinese medicine, radial pulse readings are taken at the wrist on both hands, with each of the viscera (yin) and bowel (yang) organs corresponding with a different section on either the left or right wrist. There are 28 different pulse qualities which together help the skilled physician discern the nature and location of the disease.

ANXIETY/WORRY: While healthy in moderation, constant anxiety can lead to symptoms of depression and obsessive/compulsive-type behavioural patterns.

GRIEF: Sadness and grief (when appropriately expressed) are healthy and normal reactions to life events. However, unresolved grief can injure the lungs and large intestine, the organs associated with the metal element. Poor, shallow breathing or the holding back of proper elimination are symptoms associated with excessive grief and worry.

FEAR: Fear can be either a cause or consequence of a water imbalance. Any illness affecting the bladder or kidneys can give rise to a fearful feeling, while fear itself is a protective element of survival. When in extreme it can injure the organs causing a range of problems from bedwetting to kidney stones and bladder infections.

Tongue diagnosis is also very important in Chinese medicine. The tongue is a microcosm of the internal organs with each section representing a specific organ (e.g. the tip of the tongue relates to the heart; the centre to the spleen and stomach). The tongue is observed for its colour, shape, moisture and coating. For example, a very red tongue tip indicates excessive heat in the heart (indicative of anxiety, palpitations and poor sleep) while a thick, yellow coating in the centre of the tongue is a sign of damp heat in the stomach and spleen (associated with bloating or gas and loose stools).

In Chinese medicine the fundamental root of disease can be described as an imbalance between yin and yang or an inability to return to balance. The key to effective treatment rests in identifying the location of the problem or disease, assessing its strength in relation to the person's overall strength, and using therapeutic measures to specifically address the disharmony. Patients are traditionally encouraged to "sweat out" a fever as this helps expel pathogens from the body. Similarly, coughs are not traditionally suppressed with cough medicine but rather seen as the body's positive means of expelling impurities.

Acupuncture

When *Qi* is disrupted the job of the acupuncturist is to nudge it back to equilibrium by inserting needles at specific acupoints along the meridians and pulsing the body with a low electric current to free blocked energy. Although Western scientists remain sceptical about exactly how acupuncture works, they know in certain situations it produces measurable changes in the brain.

Acupuncture gained official worldwide recognition in 1979 when the World Health Organization (WHO) issued a list of health conditions appropriate for acupuncture treatment including stress, headaches and migraines, female fertility, pregnancy-induced nausea, menstrual cramps, morning sickness, constipation, ulcers, tennis elbow, insomnia and general muscle pain. In the United States, the Food and Drug Administration (FDA) now considers acupuncture a viable alternative to conventional medicine.

There are approximately 365 acupuncture or acupoints along the body's main energy channels with many more on the lesser ones. Depending on the medical diagnosis,

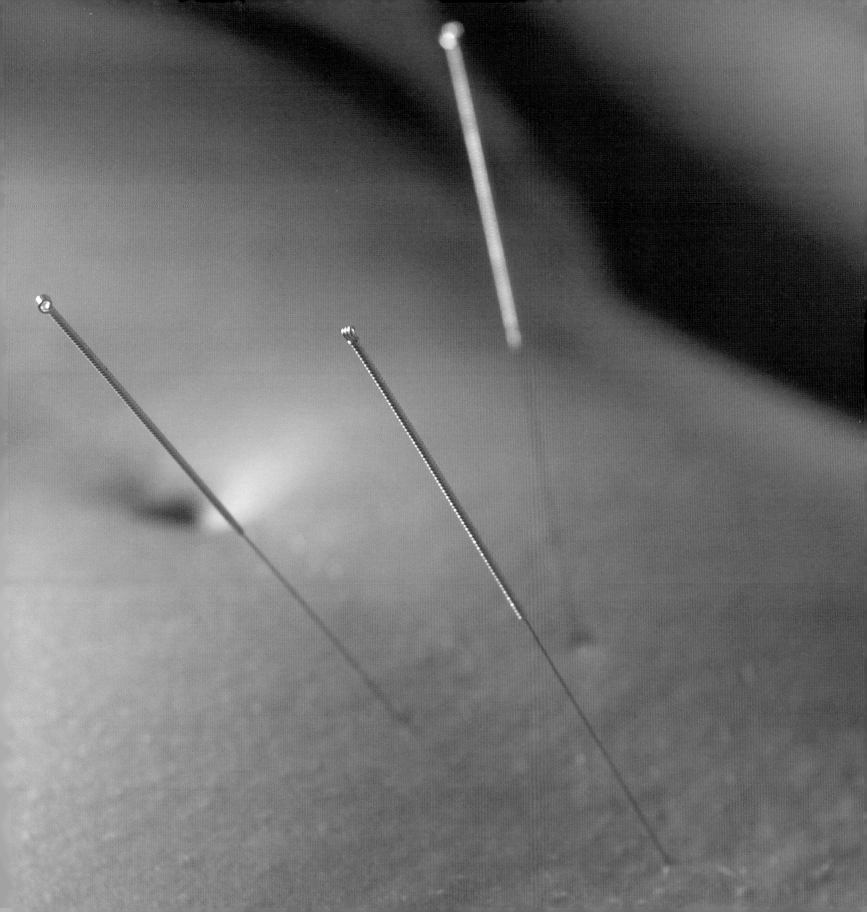

specific acupoints will be selected for treatment. Interestingly, men have more sensory receptors in their skin than women (hence the reason they feel more pain). As they tend to have a stronger response to acupuncture than women, often a more gentle approach is taken by the trained acupuncturist when treating men.

In recent years acupuncture has won many converts in the West including celebrities such as Kate Moss and Geri Halliwell; it has even featured in popular American television series including *Sex & The City* and *Friends*. Its one great advantage over Western medicine is that it does no harm; unlike drugs and surgery it has virtually no side-effects. Normally the response is gradual with symptoms sometimes worsening before marked improvement is noted. Acupuncture is also used in skincare, to firm and uplift the face and delay the signs of ageing.

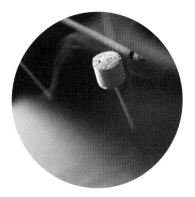

Moxibustion

Moxa is a dried form of a herb commonly known as mugwort *(Follium artemisiae)*. When applied to the acupoints, via an indirect cauterization or burning technique, its warming and invigorating properties penetrate the skin, activating the meridians and clearing blockages. The most common form of moxa used today is the moxa stick, a compressed moxa leaf resembling a small cigar which when lit is held above the skin to warm the acupoint. Alternatively it can be applied directly to the acupuncture needle to clear blocked energy.

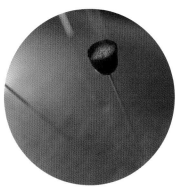

Cupping

An ancient form of therapeutic massage, cupping has become hugely popular recently because of its benefits in moving stagnant *Qi* and invigorating the system. Gwyneth Paltrow is a firm advocate who has been photographed at public events displaying the telltale circular marks left by the treatment on her back.

The ancient Taoists' hollow animal horns or bamboo have been replaced by glass light-bulb-shaped jars. These are fixed on various points in the body, using a pump to create a vacuum. The suction pulls the skin upwards within the jar, bringing a flow of blood and *Qi* to the area. Cups can be moved along specific areas of the body, creating friction. Cupping is successfully used for the relief of arthritic pain and dysmenorrhoea and is often practised in conjunction with acupuncture and massage.

Traditional Chinese Medicine and You

"Respect your body—without feelings of respect what is there to distinguish men from beasts?"

—Confucius (c. 550-478BC)

One of the greatest advantages of Chinese medicine is its comprehensive approach to health and disease prevention. This is especially important for the modern woman, whose role in creating and sustaining balanced and healthy lives for herself and her family is more complex now than ever before. With partner, children, parents, work and finances all vying for her time it becomes increasingly difficult to maintain balance and control. Stress becomes an inevitable consequence. Unresolved chronic stress causes serious *Qi* stagnation and is the root cause of many of the health problems experienced today.

Another pertinent issue for many women is the relative importance of rest and exercise. To the Chinese, exercise and rest are seen as yin/yang aspects and, to avoid burn-out, must be balanced against one another and the person's overall health and age. When we are young our bodies are at their peak and high-impact sport comes easily. However, as we age, although mental resources strengthen, physical condition changes and balance becomes more difficult to achieve. This is where lower impact exercises like *tai chi* and yoga come into their own as they encourage the smooth flow of *Qi* and blood through the body. Although higher impact sports can still be performed by older women they must be complemented with adequate recovery and relaxation.

Here are some of the questions a Chinese medical doctor would ask to gain an insight into a person's wellbeing:

⊛ **Are you constantly tired with no energy?**
⊛ **Do you have trouble sleeping at night?**
⊛ **Do you constantly think about food and eating?**
⊛ **Do you do high-impact exercise more than three times each week?**

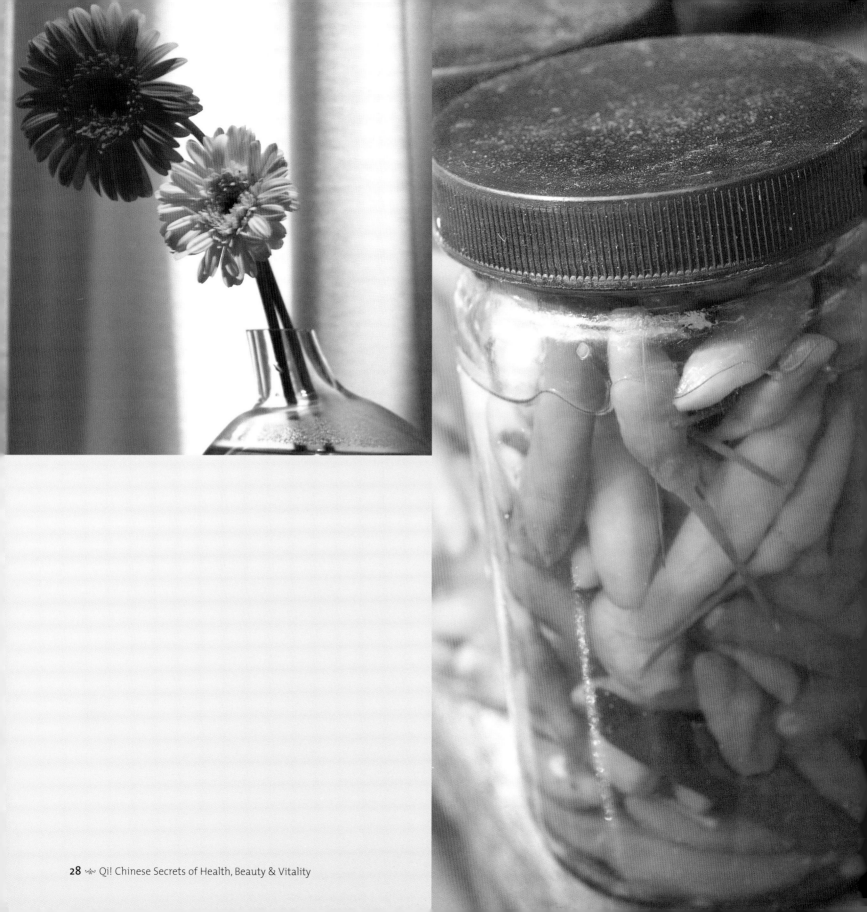

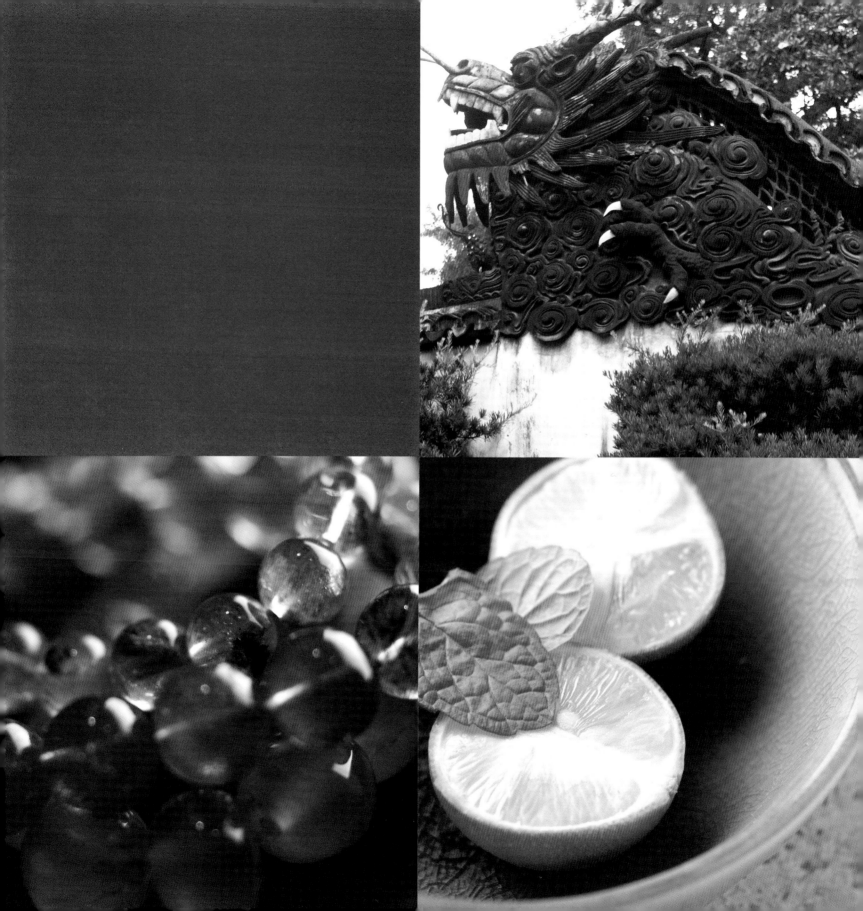

- ⚜ Are you always trying to lose weight even though you generally eat a "healthy" diet?
- ⚜ When choosing foods do you look for lower fat, lower calorie options?
- ⚜ Do you crave carbohydrates like breads, rice, pasta and potatoes?
- ⚜ Do you have ongoing digestive problems such as bloating, heartburn or irregular bowel function?
- ⚜ Are you often tired and/or suffer from headaches after eating?
- ⚜ Do you constantly feel that although you are not "sick", you are not as well as you could be?
- ⚜ Do you suffer from premenstrual symptoms/tension for at least three days a month?
- ⚜ Are your nails brittle and do they break easily?
- ⚜ Do you worry excessively and feel constantly stressed?
- ⚜ Have you become increasingly moody and cranky?
- ⚜ Have you tried to stop smoking but just can't?

If you answered "yes" to three or more of these, then working with Chinese medicine is an investment in your body which could yield far-reaching and unexpected benefits. Once you become familiar with its principles, you will discover them everywhere—from work to personal life; in people's personalities; your menstrual cycle; even the external seasons. These interwoven cycles define the dynamic of our lives—multifaceted, interconnected and perpetually in motion.

Chinese medicine is about recognizing and identifying patterns in your life and learning how to make your body work for you. If, for example, you are prone to stress-related headaches, by making some simple changes (like adjusting your exercise routine or your diet), your headaches will ease. Once you start to understand what your body needs to be its best you can wholeheartedly embrace the benefits of Traditional Chinese Medicine. The following chapters offer easy, practical ways to successfully intergrate the principles of TCM into modern life.

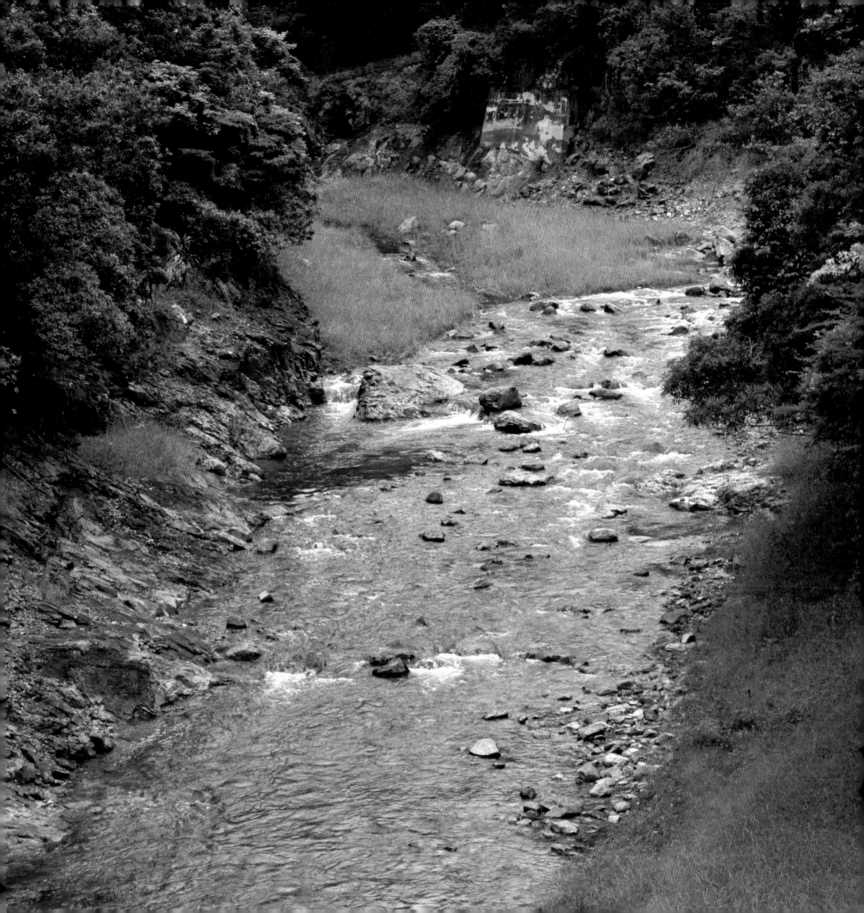

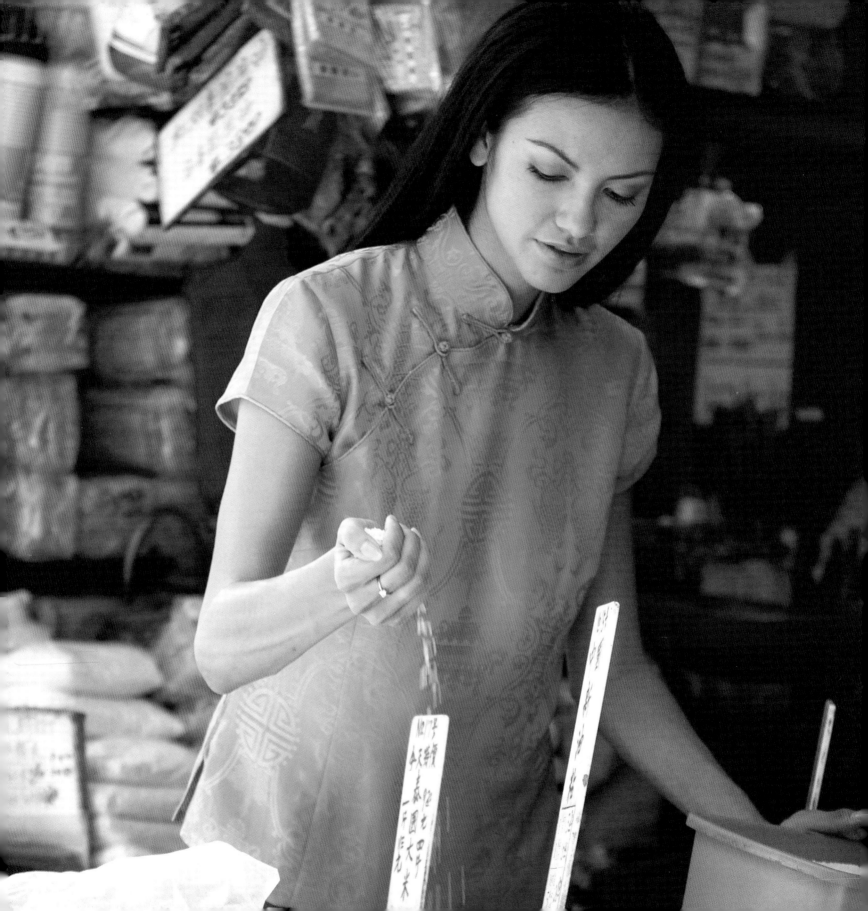

CHAPTER 2

Eating for Health:
food, herbs and tonics

"Food and drink are relied upon to nurture life. But if one does not know that the natures of substances may be opposed to each other and one consumes them altogether indiscriminately, the vital organs will be thrown out of harmony and disastrous consequences will soon arise. Therefore, those who wish to nurture their lives must carefully avoid doing such damage to themselves."

— Chia Ming, *Essential Knowledge for Eating and Drinking* (1368)

Nutrition and the power food has to harm or heal is one of the fastest growing Western sciences. Yet it is a concept that has been the cornerstone of Traditional Chinese Medicine (TCM) for centuries.

In Western thinking foods are considered for their nutritional value—the amounts of protein, carbohydrate, vitamins and minerals they contain. Although nutritional value is not completely irrelevant to the Chinese, to them foods are considered primarily for their bioenergetic natures—their energies, flavours and actions on organs once inside the body. The ultimate objective in personalizing diets Chinese-style is achieving the fine balance between yin and yang. This is done by harmonizing the five energies (natures), five flavours, the seasons and the nature of foods.

The golden rule in Chinese medicine is: "weak function: stimulate; hyperactive function: calm and sedate".

In Chinese medicine all foods can be described as "warm/stimulating", "cool/calming" or "neutral" depending on their effects once inside the body. If the body's internal energy is tired and sluggish (i.e. yin in nature), stimulating foods activate the body's yang thereby increasing energy levels. Alternatively, calming foods soothe and de-stress the organs making them the perfect complement to excess yang, while neutral foods like rice have little influence in either direction. To the Chinese maintaining this delicate internal harmony is the key to health and balance.

How foods are cooked has a powerful effect on their subsequent actions in the body,

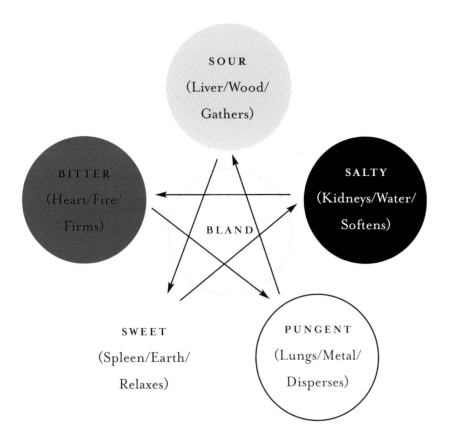

with warm and cooked foods being more easily available to the organs. Frying, roasting, grilling, smoking and spicing stimulate the internal organs while steaming, boiling and stewing calm and soothe.

Food Flavours

"The five flavours enter the body through the mouth and are stored in the intestines and stomach . . . When activity is harmonious and saliva and body fluids are mutually supportive, this gives rise to life and animation."

—*Yellow Emperor's Classic of Internal Medicine* (220BC)

The ancient Chinese classified foods into six flavour groups: sour, bitter, sweet, pungent

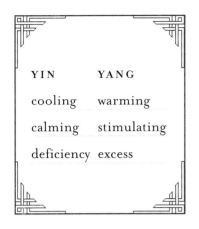

YIN	YANG
cooling	warming
calming	stimulating
deficiency	excess

and salty (associated with the Five Elements) and bland (a neutral flavour). Take the pungent flavour of wasabi (Japanese horseradish) or an onion, for instance. Associated with the metal element and lung organ, pungent-flavoured foods open the nose and mouth, clearing blocked sinuses and relieving the symptoms of colds and flu. However, while each flavour benefits a specific organ, overeating one type of food may harm another organ. Thus sour food benefits the liver but too much may hurt the spleen (which in turn influences the kidneys, and so on). As with other facets of the Chinese system, moderation is key.

Food Natures

The nature or inherent temperature of foods determines their effects once inside the body and can be defined as hot, warm, cool, cold and neutral. For example, eating foods with a hot nature or energy like chilli peppers induces a feeling of warmth. Conversely tea (although generally taken hot) has a cool energy. As a general rule, root vegetables are warming, leafy greens cooling, fruit is neutral, meat is neutral to warm, and seafood is cooling.

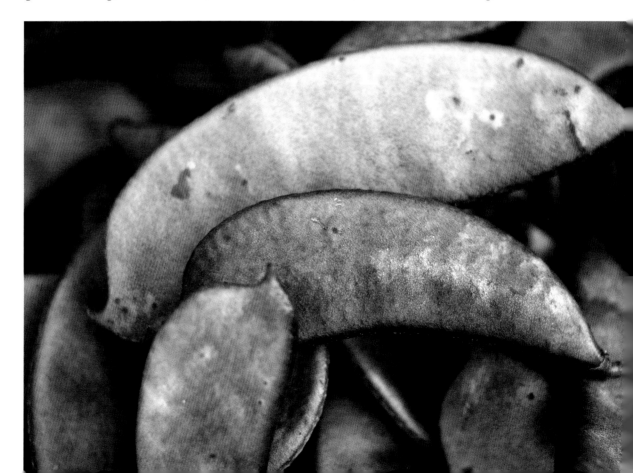

NATURE OF FOODS

COOL/CALMING	NEUTRAL	WARM/STIMULATING
American ginseng	Abalone	Anise
Apples	Adzuki Beans	Bell peppers
Asparagus	Almonds	Black sesame seeds
Bamboo shoots	Apricots	Butter
Bananas	Beef	Broad/horse beans
Barley	Beetroot	Cauliflower
Beansprouts	Black fungus	Cashews
Broccoli	Black/soy beans	Chestnuts
Button mushrooms	Bread	Cherries
Carrots	Brown rice	Chicken/Duck
Celery	Cheese	Chilli peppers
Chicory	Cabbage	Chocolate
Chinese cabbage	Chickpeas	Coconut milk and meat
Crab	Crab apples	Coffee
Egg white	Eggs	Corn
Fennel	Endive	Dates
Fish (white)	Grapes	Eel
Frogs' legs	Honey	Eggplant
Grapefruit	Licorice (Chinese)	Egg yolk
Green tea	Milk (cow's)	Figs
Ham	Oats	Fried foods
Hops	Papaya	Gingko
Kelp/seaweed	Pasta	Guavas

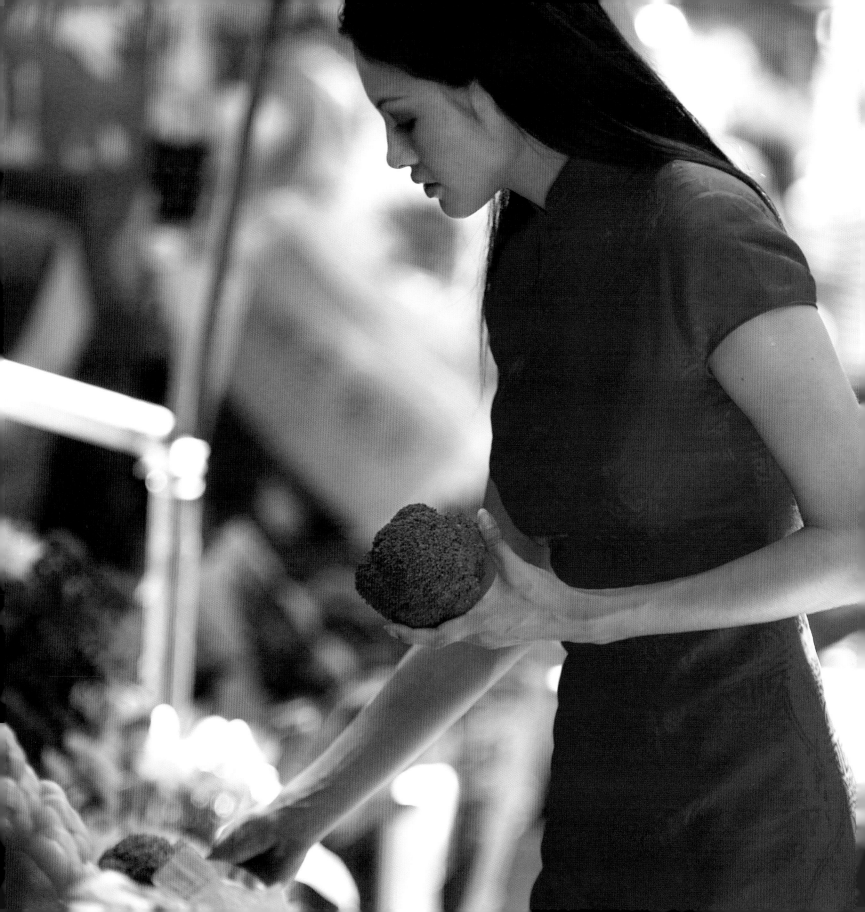

NATURE OF FOODS (CONTINUED)

COOL/CALMING	NEUTRAL	WARM/STIMULATING
Lettuce	Pineapples	Kidney beans
Loquats	Pinto beans	Korean ginseng
Lotus leaves and roots	Pork	Lamb
Melons	Potatoes	Leeks
Oranges	Salmon	Lemons/limes
Oysters	Sardines	Lentils
Peanuts (raw)	Seaweed	Longans
Pears	Soybeans	Mandarin orange peel
Plantain	Squid	Mussels
Plums	Wheat/wheatgerm	Onions/scallions
Radishes	White rice	Peaches
Rhubarb	White sesame seeds	Peas/snow peas
Salad greens	Trout	Peanut butter/oil
Snails	Tuna	Pickles
Soybean curd/tofu		Pumpkins
Spinach		Raspberries
Starfruit (carombola)		Red wine
Strawberries		Root vegetables
Tangerines		Sesame seed oil
Tomatoes		Shitake mushrooms
Vinegar		Sheep's milk
Water chestnuts		Sherry
Watercress		Shrimp/prawns
Yoghurt		Siberian ginseng
		Smoked meat/fish

NATURE OF FOODS (CONTINUED)

WARM/STIMULATING

Sunflower seeds

Sweet potatoes

Taro

Turkey

Venison

Walnuts

Whiskey

Winter squashes

HERBS, SPICES AND CONDIMENTS

COOL/CALMING	NEUTRAL	WARM/STIMULATING
Lemongrass	Sugar	Basil
Mint/peppermint		Bay leaf
Parsley		Black pepper
Salt		Cardamom
Vanilla		Cayenne pepper
		Cinnamon
		Clove
		Coriander
		Curry powder
		Dill
		Garlic
		Ginger
		Miso
		Nutmeg
		Oregano

NOTE: **Food energies are for foods in their raw state. Cooking alters the nature of foods.**

Eating with the Seasons

To maintain harmony with the natural world the body must match nature's cycles by working with the Five Elements and eating with the seasons. Root vegetables, being warming, are more plentiful during the colder winter months while summer is the time for light, clean food with cooling fresh fruits and leafy greens in abundance. The Liver Flush (page 79) is ideally carried out at the start of a new season as it cleanses from within, setting the body up for the months ahead.

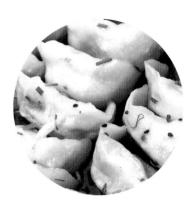

SPRING: Associated with the wood element, Spring's yang energy is abundant, characterized by nature shooting upwards. Eating to support the wood element means "clean" eating of pungent and sweet fruits and vegetables with little fat, sugar, alcohol, coffee and chemicals. It is the ideal season for detoxifying a congested liver in preparation for the hot summer months (see Fourteen-Day Cleanse, page 74). Greens are a traditional part of the spring diet in most cultures. Being plentiful and packed with chlorophyll (which absorbs energy from the sun), their use is associated with freshening, cleansing and rebuilding the body.

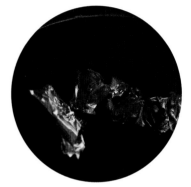

SUMMER: The fire element means energy, warmth and vitality. The body's yang *Qi* is surfacing, pores are open and sweating is the norm. Cooling and bitter fruit- and vegetable-based foods and drinks drain *Qi* downwards to quell the excess fire heat. Foods should be lightly cooked (think boiling, steaming and stir-frying) and the diet packed with cooling foods like fruits, salad greens, cucumber, lemons, limes, seeds and mint. Chicken and dairy products being more yang in nature should be restricted.

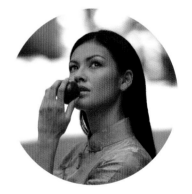

LONG SUMMER: Associated with the earth element, the long summer's heat, rain and humidity can affect the function of the heart and spleen, giving rise to increased sweating, poor appetite, bloating, heavy limbs and soft stools. Cooling foods and drinks like celery, watermelon and cucumber help reduce these symptoms and humidity-induced fluid retention.

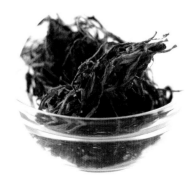

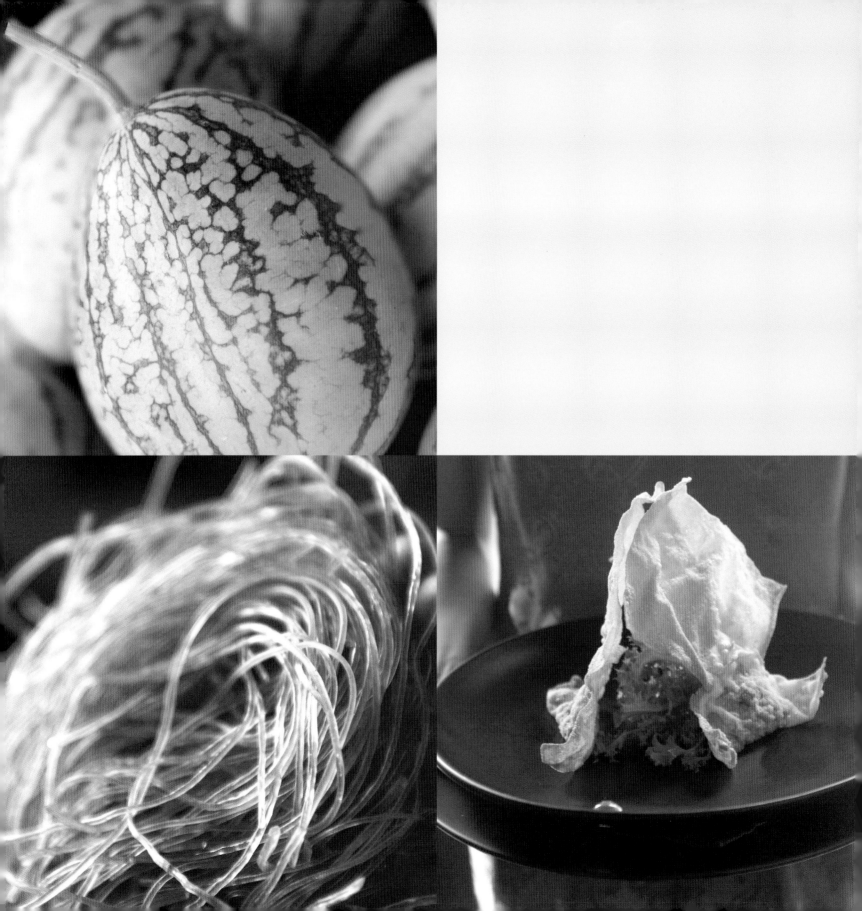

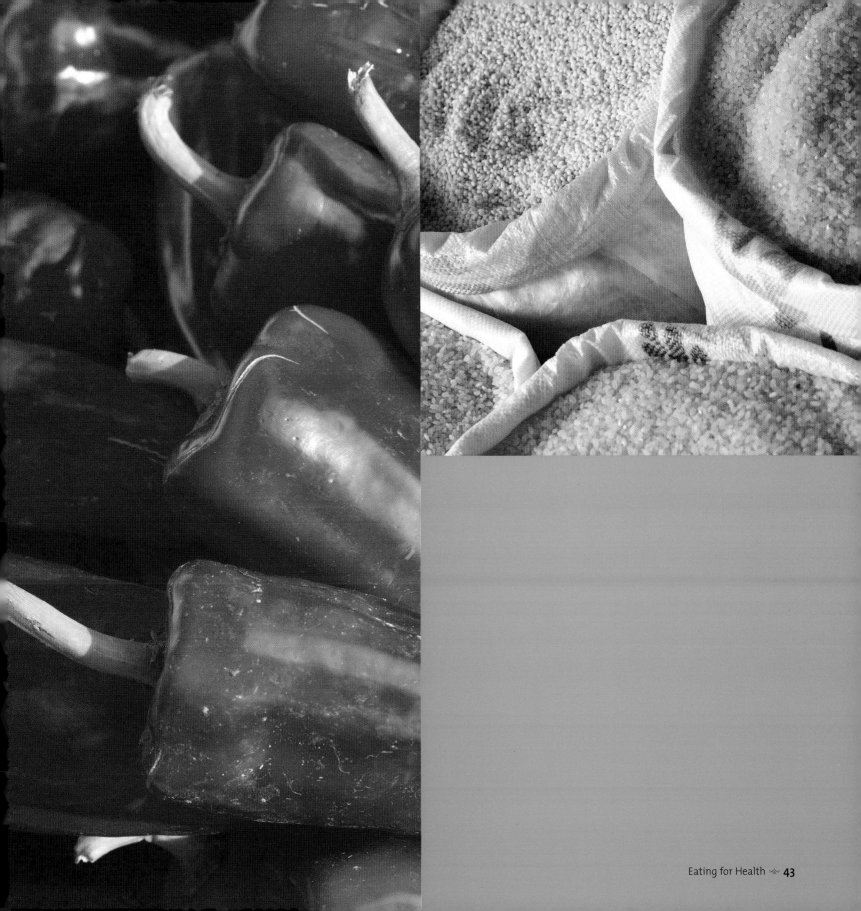

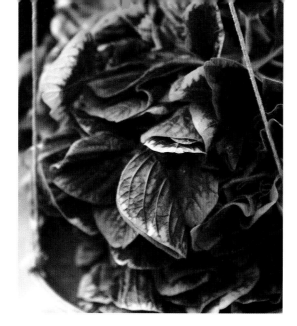
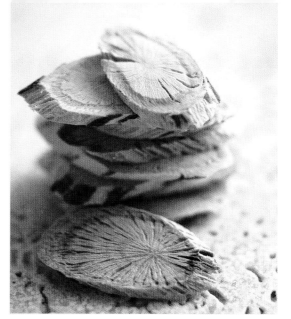

Long Summer also signifies the beginning of harvest time when nature is rich and sweet with apples, corn, grapes, tomatoes and beans.

AUTUMN: The season of ripening characterized by the metal element, Autumn is traditionally dry so the lungs need added protection to keep them healthy and moist. Hearty foods like fish, vegetables, olive oil and stronger tasting warming foods such as meat, eggs and dairy products combined with longer cooking methods (baking and roasting) help draw energy into the food to heat the body.

WINTER: Associated with the water element, Winter is the yin season of storage. It is the time when *Qi* needs most protection and warmer clothes are worn (especially in colder climates). The water element's vegetables and fruits spread outwards like waves or ripples (think seaweed and mushrooms), while Winter's flavour, salt, penetrates the kidneys and bladder, regulating water balance in the body. Traditionally a time for soups, stews and casseroles, Winter meals require garlic, ginger and cayenne pepper to add warmth to the body. Cooked whole grains (especially millet and buckwheat which are less starchy) served with lentils or beans are excellent winter staples.

WOOD/SPRING

Fresh fruits, green vegetables,
asparagus, corn, wheat, celery, cucumber,
berries, lemons, sour plums, yoghurt,
limes, pickles, brown rice, nuts,
seeds and dandelion

FIRE/SUMMER

Grains, broccoli, spinach,
apricots, peaches, cherries, salad greens,
cucumber, lemons, limes,
cayenne, ginger, lemongrass,
mint and seeds

EARTH/LONG SUMMER

Apples, corn, grapes, watermelon,
tomatoes, celery, cucumber, beans, eggs,
fish and poultry

WATER/WINTER

Baked and roasted dishes,
soups, stews, meats, turnips, seaweed,
mushrooms, squashes, melons and
salt (sea salt, soy sauce)

METAL/AUTUMN

Root vegetables (potatoes,
yams, squashes, carrots, onions),
spinach, nuts, beans, seeds, garlic, ginger,
meats, dairy products (including eggs),
mangoes and bananas

The TCM of Vitamins and Minerals

The relationship between different foods and *Qi* can be further explained by the actions on specific body organs and emotions of vitamin and mineral substances which naturally occur in food (and are also taken as supplements). According to *The Tao of Healthy Eating* (2002), these actions (which all help improve *Qi* flow) are as follows.

VITAMINS

Vitamin A: Supplements and clears heat from the blood and brightens the eyes.

Vitamin B1: Fortifies the liver and spleen; dries "dampness"; stops pain.

Vitamin B2: Nourishes the liver, stomach and kidneys.

Vitamin B3: Soothes the liver and stomach; clears heat.

Vitamin B5: Fortifies the liver and spleen, soothes the stomach; clears heat; eases depression.

Vitamin B6: Fortifies the liver; clears heat from the stomach and damp heat from the gall-bladder; eases depression. Harmonizes the wood and earth elements.

Vitamin B12: Nourishes the blood and stops bleeding.

Vitamin B15: Quickens the blood.

Biotin: Nourishes the blood; soothes the liver; strengthens the heart; calms the spirit.

Choline: Nourishes the blood; reduces wind; strengthens the sinews and bones; moistens the intestines.

Folic Acid: Nourishes the blood; harmonizes the liver; calms the foetus and the spirit.

Inositol: Nourishes the blood; moistens the intestines; calms the spirit.

PABA (para-aminobenzoic acid): Supplements the liver and kidneys; moistens the intestines; dispels wind; helps stool flow; blackens hair; retards ageing.

Vitamin C: Stops bleeding; resolves toxins; clears heat from the heart; calms the spirit.

Vitamin D: Supplements the kidneys; strengthens sinews and bones; brightens the eyes; invigorates yang; soothes the foetus.

Vitamin E: Nourishes the blood; strengthens sinews and bones; supplements yang.

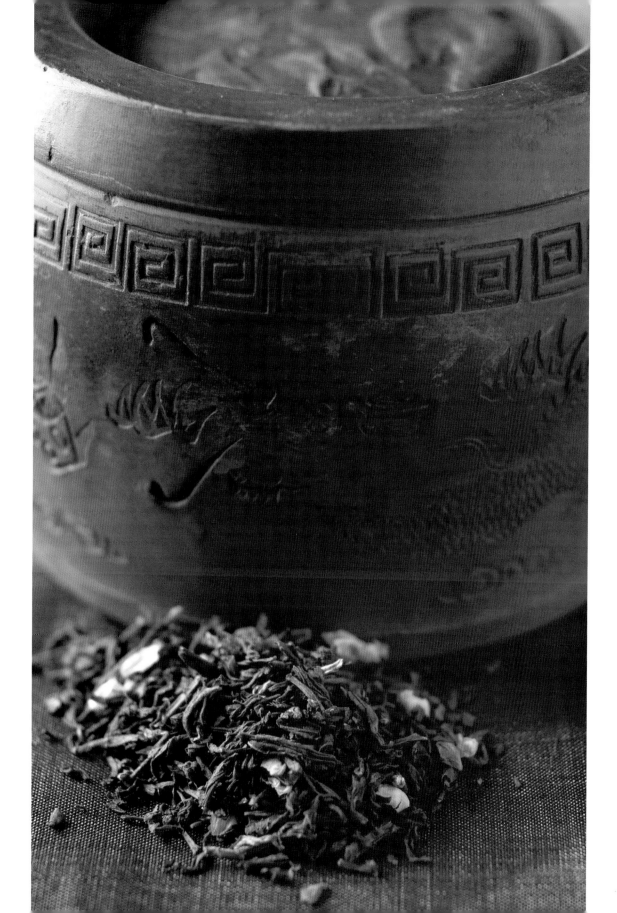

Vitamin K: Aids the lungs and large intestine; stops bleeding.

Bioflavonoids: Quickens the blood; clears heat from the blood; stops bleeding.

Beta-Carotene: Courses the liver; resolves toxins; disperses stagnations and accumulations; combats cancer.

MINERALS

Calcium: Astringes yin and suppresses yang; strengthens the bones; promotes new tissue generation; absorbs acid; stops pain.

Chromium: Fortifies the spleen; supplements the blood.

Cobalt: Supplements the blood.

Copper: Fortifies the spleen; eliminates damp heat.

Fluorine: Supplements the kidneys; strengthens the bones and teeth; enriches yin.

Iodine: Courses the liver; scatters nodulation; clears heat.

Iron: Cools and quickens the blood; clears heat.

Magnesium: Astringes yin and suppresses yang; absorbs acid; stops pain; calms the spirit.

Manganese: Nourishes the liver; enriches the kidneys; strengthens the sinews and bones; sharpens the hearing.

Molybdenum: Cools and nourishes the blood; clears heat; enriches yin.

Phosphorus: Supplements the kidneys; strengthens the sinews and bones; enriches yin.

Potassium: Fortifies the spleen; expels pus; dispels wind; eliminates damp heat.

Selenium: Astringes yin and suppresses yang; brightens the eyes; calms the spirit.

Silica: Supplements the kidneys and strengthens the bones.

Silicon: Supplements the liver and kidneys and strengthens the sinews and bones.

Sodium: Supplements the liver and kidneys; softens hardness; scatters nodulation.

Sulphur: Supplements the kidneys; blackens the hair; benefits the skin; warms yang.

Zinc: Nourishes the liver and kidneys; strengthens the bones; brightens the eyes.

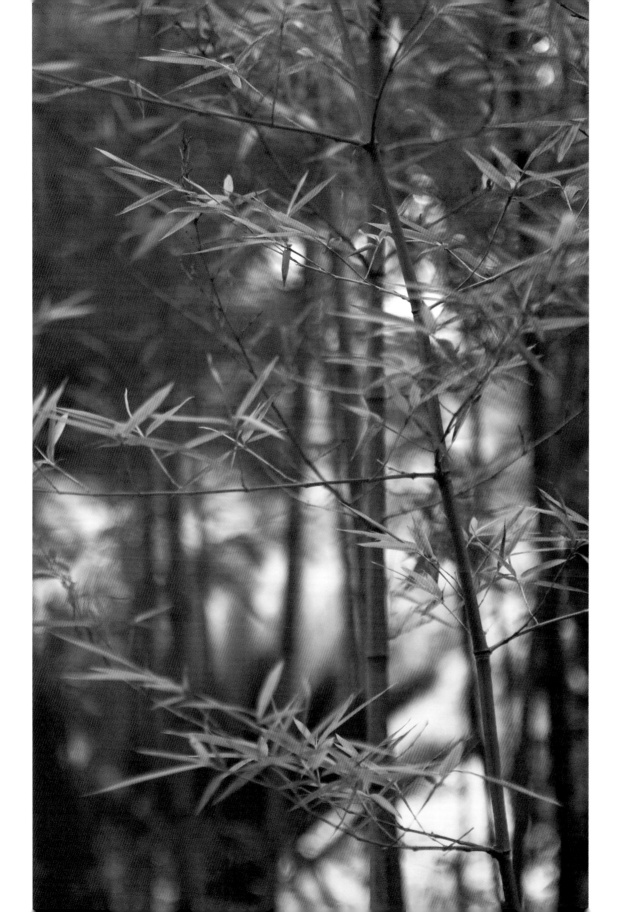

What Foods Should I Eat?

Although each of us is an individual, Chinese medicine maintains that regardless of your make-up, eating with the seasons is essential to ensure that hot summer weather is complemented with cooling yin foods and that the cold of winter is complemented with yang's internal warmth. In tropical climates where heat is constant, foods should be primarily light and lean with the emphasis on fresh leafy greens, fruits, leaner meats and fish with less dairy products and refined carbohydrates.

The bulk of the traditional Chinese diet comprises unrefined carbohydrates and fibre-rich vegetables with less animal protein, refined sugars, oils and fats. Cooking food is essential to assist digestion by starting the breakdown process outside the body. Although the Chinese drink water, it is never cold. To them, cold food or drinks slow digestion; if too many raw and cold foods are eaten more energy is required to break them down. Chewing food is extremely important too. Just as herbs and spices need to be crushed to liberate their aromas and goodness, the more food is chewed the more available it is to the body.

Breakfast literally breaks the night's fast and a large glass of warm(ish) water helps replenish fluids and sets the digestive system up for the day. Fruits are generally not encouraged at breakfast as they have a cooling nature that slows digestion (especially when used straight from the fridge). However, red fruits like papaya, raspberries[*], red grapes, pink grapefruit, strawberries and watermelon eaten at room temperature are a stimulating start. See pages 54-58 for suggested breakfast recipes. Skipping meals is not encouraged as regular meals keep the digestive system working steadily.

Eating large meals late in the evening can lead to indigestion and stomach discomfort, not to mention fitful sleep. In Chinese thinking this is due to stomach *Qi* burnout. By sim-

High Protein/Low Carbohydrate Diets
Diets such as Atkins, The Zone and Body for Life are currently very popular in the West. However, traditional Chinese wisdom states that high protein diets (packed with meat, eggs and cheese) are warming to the body so would only be recommended for cool, yin types who need added warmth. A high protein diet would make a hot, yang person even more unbalanced. Carbohydrates (e.g. rice and wheat) have neutral energy. However, the main problem with wheat (the principal carbohydrate eaten in the West) is that it produces phlegm and in some people can lead to fluid retention and bloating. Regardless of food type, overall balance is key.

[*]*Chinese medicine practitioners believe that eating unripe (green) raspberries raises body temperature, particularly in the genital area, and is beneficial for women unable to conceive due to "cold in the uterus". Making raspberries part of your diet also reputably improves the skin's appearance and helps prevent hair from greying.*

ply eating earlier (i.e. two to three hours before bed) and eating less—following the "75 per cent" rule (the stomach being half full with food, one quarter with liquid and one quarter empty)—that sluggish feeling can disappear and health and sleep patterns may improve.

Water is essential especially in hotter climates. However, forcing eight glasses of water into the body can be as detrimental as not drinking any. Listen to your body. In warmer climates cooling drinks like grape or watermelon juice and unfermented tea (great for the skin too) are all-round thirst quenchers. Cooler weather dictates more warming fluids.

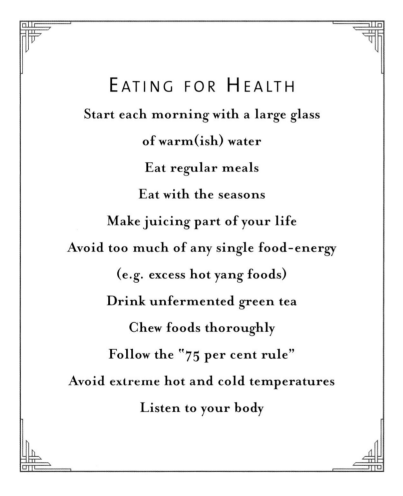

EATING FOR HEALTH

Start each morning with a large glass

of warm(ish) water

Eat regular meals

Eat with the seasons

Make juicing part of your life

Avoid too much of any single food-energy

(e.g. excess hot yang foods)

Drink unfermented green tea

Chew foods thoroughly

Follow the "75 per cent rule"

Avoid extreme hot and cold temperatures

Listen to your body

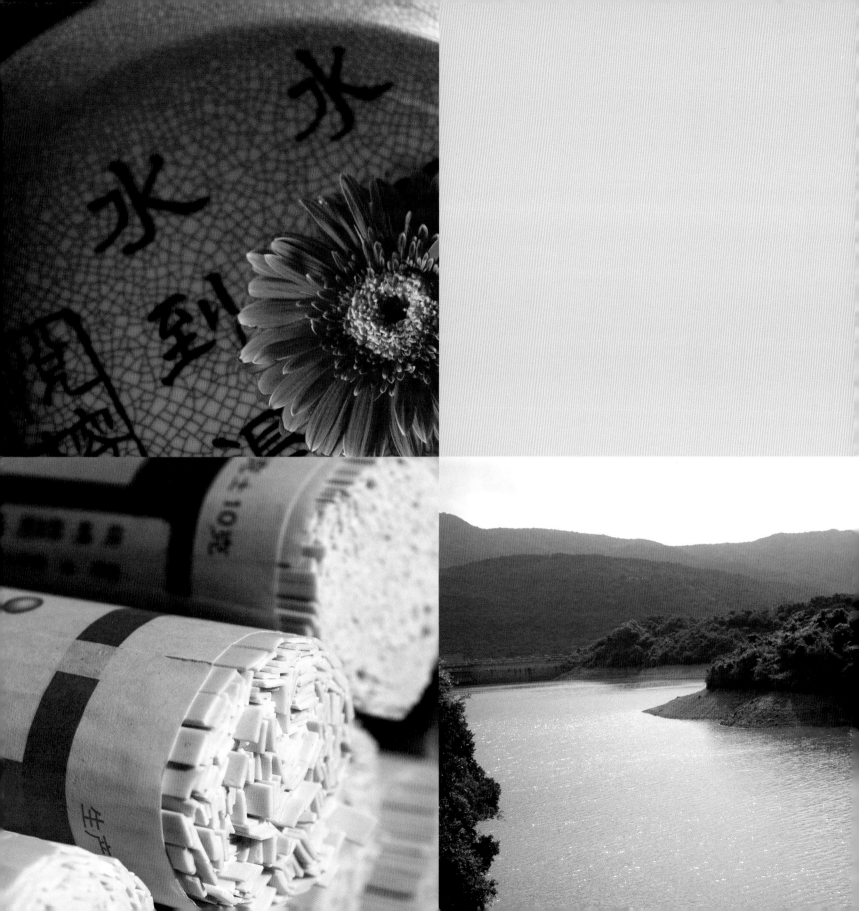

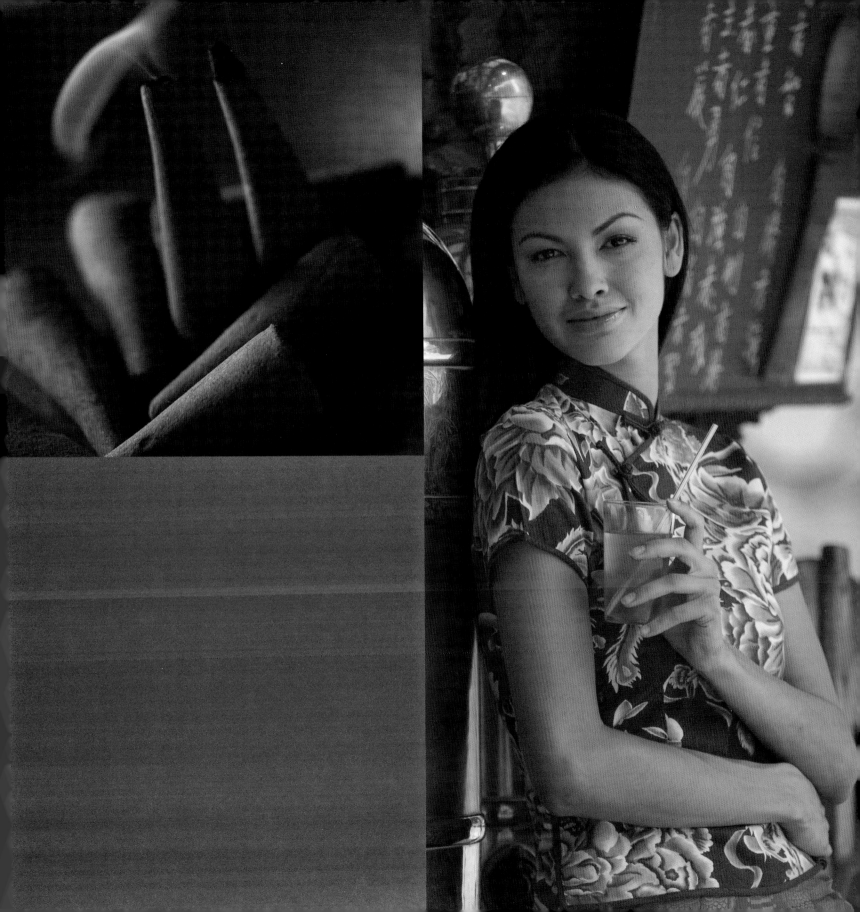

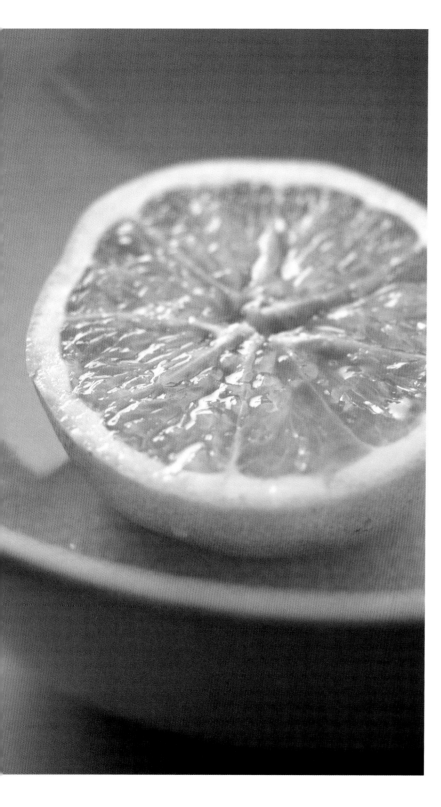

Seasonal Power Breakfasts

(All recipes serve one person unless stated)

Spring: Bircher Muesli

2 tbsp oat flakes (or combination of oat, rye or wheat)

1 apple/firm pear, grated

Handful of soaked raisins

$^1/_2$ lemon

2 tbsp plain low fat yoghurt

1 tbsp chopped nuts (e.g. almonds or brazil nuts)

1 tsp honey or powdered ginger

Other preferred fresh fruits can also be added

    e.g. strawberries, raspberries, prunes, apricots

    and bananas

Soak the flakes and raisins overnight in a little water or pure fruit juice. Before eating add the grated apple or pear with a squeeze of lemon juice, the yoghurt and other seasonal fruits. Drizzle with honey if desired and sprinkle with chopped nuts and ginger.

Summer: Mango and Orange Coulée

2 medium mangoes

2 large juice oranges

1 tsp cornstarch

$^3/_4$ tsp freshly grated root ginger

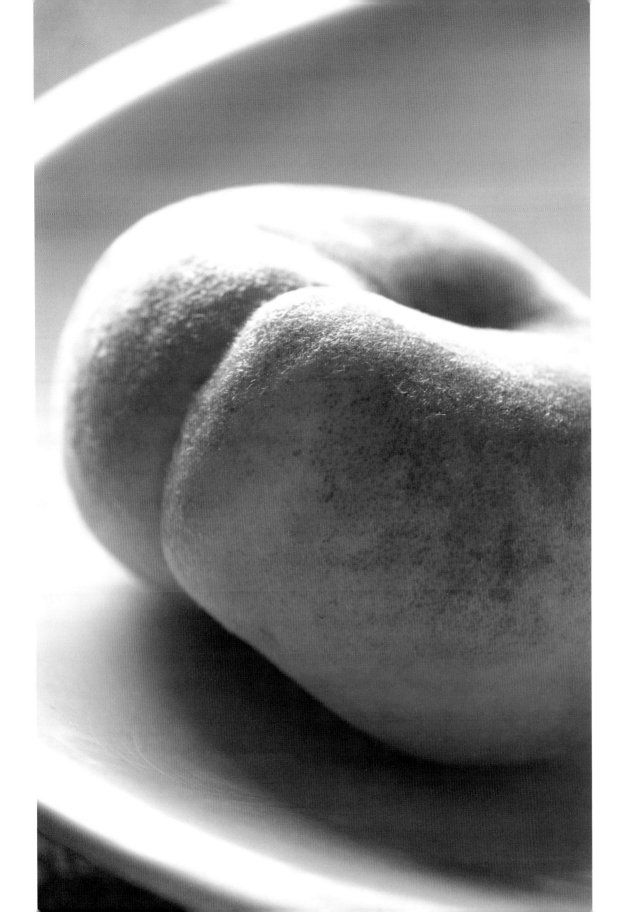

Peel and cut mangoes into large chunks. Pit the oranges and pulp into a small bowl and add the cornstarch, ginger and salt. Pour into a heated pot and stir over a medium heat until it starts to thicken. Add the mango and cook for a few minutes before serving.

Long Summer: Berry Smoothie

2 cups assorted berries (strawberries, raspberries, blackberries or other seasonal fruits)

$^3/_4$ cup soy milk

50g/2oz low fat fruit yoghurt (with active bacterial cultures)

2 ice cubes

Combine all ingredients in blender and purée. Add a handful of sunflower, flax or sesame seeds if desired and drink immediately.

Autumn: Walnut, Apple and Pear Stew

3 red apples

3 ripe pears

$^1/_2$ carrot

1 cup water

$^1/_2$ tsp cinnamon

A dollop of natural yoghurt (with active bacterial cultures)

10 roasted walnuts

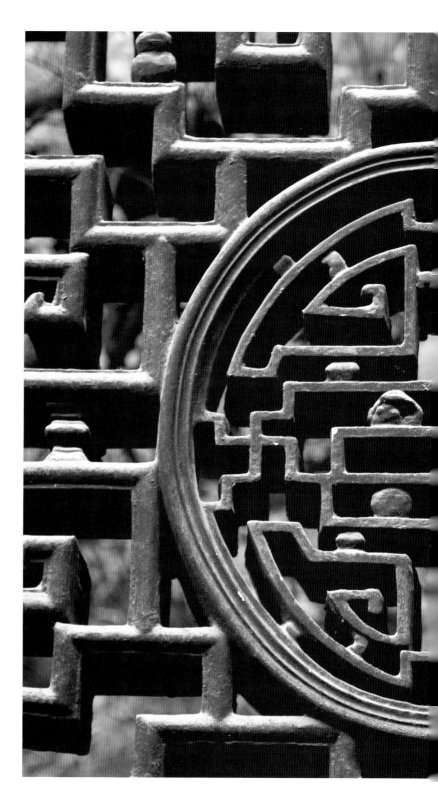

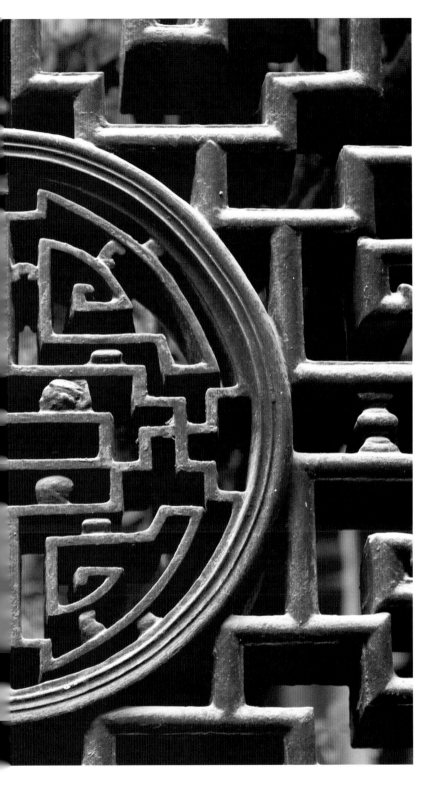

Peel and core the apples, pears and carrot and cut into 1.25cm (half-inch) chunks. Add water and cinnamon, cover and cook over medium heat for 20 minutes until soft. Remove from heat and serve warm with chopped walnuts and natural yoghurt.

Winter: Warming Congee

(4 servings)

1.5kg (3.5 to 4lb) chicken cut into serving pieces
    with giblets (excluding liver)

10 cups water

3 tbsp Chinese rice wine or sherry

3 slices of fresh ginger,
    about 0.5cm (0.75 inches) thick

3 spring onions, halved crosswise and smashed
    with side of a heavy knife

$^{1}/_{2}$ tsp salt

$^{1}/_{2}$ cup long-grain rice

Bring chicken and water to the boil in a large saucepan, skimming the froth. Add the rice wine, ginger, spring onions and salt and simmer uncovered for 20 minutes or until breast meat is cooked through. Remove chicken breasts, cool and tear into shreds.

Add rice to the stock mixure. Bring to the boil and stir. Reduce heat to low and simmer, covered, for about 20-30 minutes, stirring frequently. Congee will continue to thicken as it stands so thin with water if necessary. Season with salt and serve topped with chicken shreds and thinly sliced spring onions.

Summer: Cooling Grape Juice

Grape juice made from dark grapes is wonderful for replenishing yin fluids and cooling summer's heat. Grape ice cubes can also be made by pouring the juice into an ice-cube tray. Add a few cubes to sparkling water or summer lemonade for a taste of yin's cool.

Winter: Warming Ginger Tea

(6 servings)

$1/2$ cup thinly sliced fresh ginger

6 cups water

Honey to taste

Simmer ginger in water for about 20 minutes (more for stronger tea). Add honey to taste. Pour into a teapot using a sieve to strain. Serve garnished with lemon.

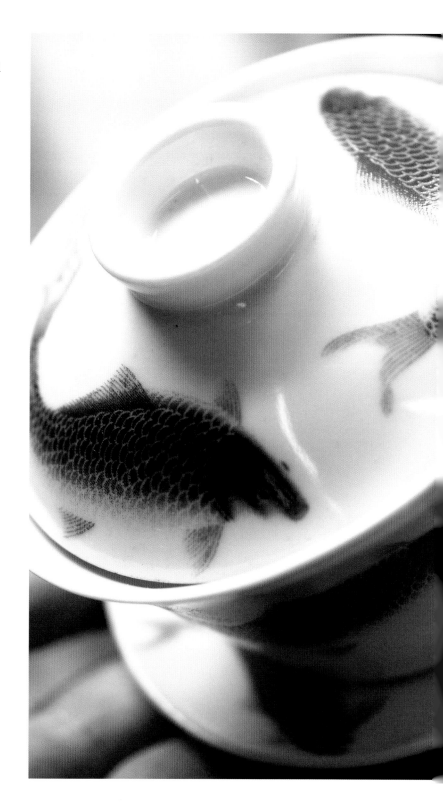

Chinese Medicinal Herbs and Tonics

"A truly good physician first finds out the cause of the illness and having found that he first tries to cure it by food. Only when food fails does he prescribe medication."

—Sun Si-mo, *Precious Recipes* (c.581-622AD)

CHINESE HERBS

As with foods, Chinese herbs are rated according to their energies, flavours and nature once inside the body. Extremely hot or warm herbs are yang, cold and cool herbs are yin, while those equally balanced are "neutral". Additionally, the same herb can have opposing actions depending on how it is eaten. For example, ginger dried in the sun is far hotter and more pungent than the fresh variety. The key to using Chinese herbs is to cool down what is hot and heat what is cold, thereby maintaining that fundamental balance.

Chinese herbs are categorized according to their basic biochemical composition and medicinal effects, which together determine what herbalists call their "natural affinities". For example, herbs used for liver problems share an affinity with the liver meridian. When the herb is metabolized in the body, its energy enters the liver meridian and its therapeutic action targets the liver directly.

MEDICINAL TONICS

"With the aid of external tonics, we are better able to cultivate the internal elixir within."

—Master Hui Ssu (6th Century AD)

The category of herbs known as "tonic medicines" (*buyao*) are the most highly prized plants in the entire Chinese pharmacopoeia. While Western medicine uses drugs to treat diseases, the Chinese use tonics to boost vitality and prevent disease by nourishing *Qi*, blood, yin and/or yang. Many of these herbs (like ginseng) are fast gaining acceptance by medical experts in the West. One of the great wonders of Chinese medicine is that over the centuries it has investigated virtually every element of the earth's landscape in its quest for health and harmony. Following is an introduction to the main Chinese tonic medicines and recipes involving them.

Chinese Herbal Flavours

Sweet herbs are often used as a tonic as they warm, soothe, nourish and relax. They act on the spleen and stomach to enhance energy circulation through the body. Common sweet-tasting herbs include cinnamon, ginseng and bamboo shoots.

Bitter herbs detoxify, cool and disperse. They cleanse the blood and protect against infection. Bitter herbs include watercress and rhubarb.

Pungent herbs are acrid and spicy and their prime action is to stimulate, disperse and invigorate the system, especially the lungs and large intestine. They help open pores and encourage sweating so are ideal for treating colds and flu. Pungent herbs include ginger, mint and black pepper.

Salty herbs are used for their diuretic and softening actions primarily on the kidneys and bladder. Their softening effect is especially beneficial for treating hardened lymph nodes and constipation. Seaweed is an example.

Sour herbs absorb, refresh and stimulate digestion. They affect the liver and gallbladder primarily and are beneficial in stopping diarrhoea, bleeding and excessive perspiration. Sour herbs include lemon, crab apple, orange peel and gooseberry.

Bland (or neutral) herbs include licorice.

While each flavour denotes a specific property of the herb, many herbs have more than one flavour.

CHINESE HERBAL FORMULATIONS

The Chinese herbs most commonly prescribed—for conditions ranging from fatigue to infertility—are as formulae containing up to 20 herbs which are categorized as follows:

- ❖ 1-2 **emperor herbs (main herbs used to treat presenting symptoms)**
- ❖ 1-4 **minister herbs (herbs which assist with associated symptoms)**
- ❖ 1-3 **adjunct herbs (which direct other herbs to specific areas of the body e.g. the throat, head, skin or kidneys)**
- ❖ 1-3 **harmonizers (which reduce any harsh or toxic effects of the herbs)**

When individual herbs are mentioned in this book, they are representative of the emperor herbs in each of the formulations outlined and for maximum therapeutic effect are best taken as part of a formulation rather than on their own. In Chinese medicine, there are more than 1,100 commonly used formulae.

Generally it takes at least three months before the therapeutic effects of the herbs are noticed. Although the dosage is outlined for each formulation mentioned, it is best to consult with a Chinese medicine practitioner or herbalist before starting herbal therapy.

The formulations listed in this book have met with the highest in international GMP (Good Manufacturing Practice) standards. GMP certification assures the public that the patent formulations are made under the highest levels of hygiene and quality control, thereby guaranteeing that they are pure (free from heavy metals, pesticides, microorganisms, pharmaceuticals, artificial colours and flavours). On-site inspections are generally repeated every two years; a factory which fails to maintain full compliance with GMP codes forfeits its certification.

GINSENG

Radix panax ginseng (Chinese or Korean); ren shen

Ginseng is an extraordinarily powerful tonic stimulating the nervous and endocrine systems, thereby increasing vital energy and treating a range of deficiency states including chronic fatigue, sleep problems, weakness and anxiety. According to the *Yellow Emperor's Classic of Internal Medicine* (220BC), "Ginseng is a tonic to the five viscera, quieting the animal spirits, stabilizing the soul, preventing fear, expelling the viscous energies, brightening the eyes and improving vision, opening up the heart, benefiting the understanding, and if taken for some time, will invigorate the body and prolong life."

Although ginseng extracts and powders are now widely available, a tea of top-quality ginseng should be taken monthly, while detoxing or at the beginning of each seasonal cycle.

Ginseng Tea

(2 servings)

1 sliced ginseng root

2 cups water

Place ginseng root in a small glass jar and pour in two cups of boiling water and cover. Place this at the bottom of a larger pot with water and let the water simmer for 6-8 hours, watching water levels. (To prevent the ginseng water from boiling and the jar from breaking, place

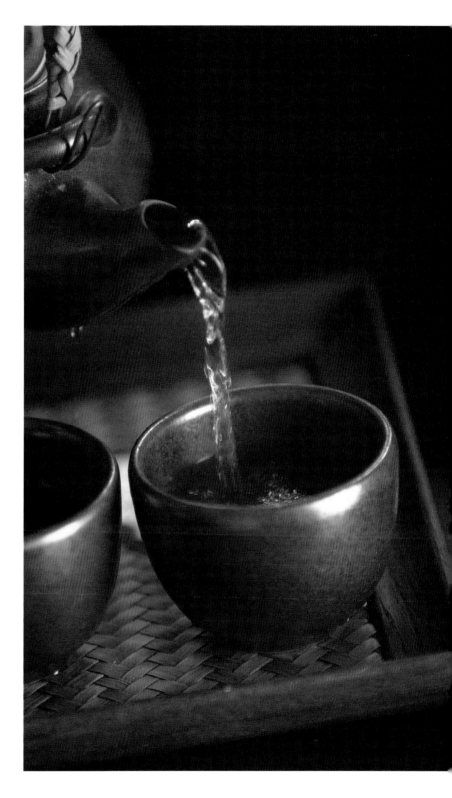

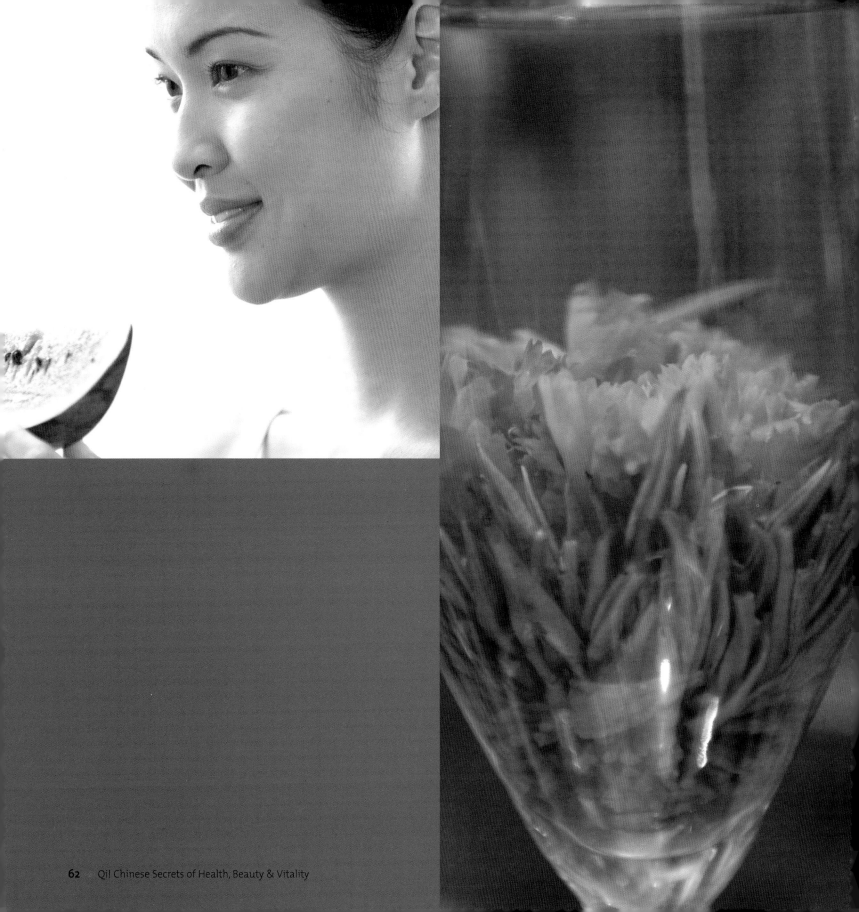

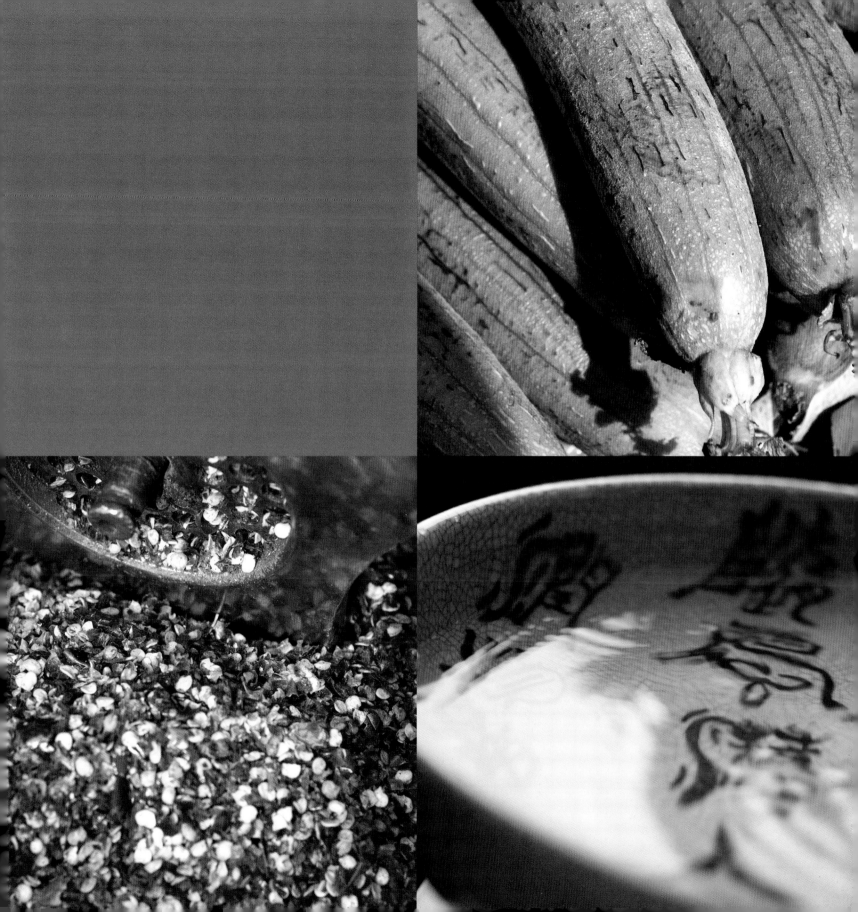

Taking Chinese Herbs

Chinese herbs can be taken in many ways, the simplest being as a tea, usually made from dried herbs (see opposite page).

Powders are ground herbs or those that have been decocted and dried into a more concentrated form. Usually the powder is mixed in warm water before drinking. Powders can also be mixed with oil or water and used externally on the skin.

Tinctures made by soaking herbs in alcohol are considered an effective means of stimulating energy and circulation. Red wine is the alcohol of choice for helping replenish post-menstrual blood loss. Liniments are prepared in the same way but used externally to treat injuries and muscular pain.

Pills are absorbed more slowly than teas, powders and tinctures and are ideal for conditions that require prolonged and slow release of the prescription.

Congees are a type of soup in which the herbs are cooked with rice until it has a porridge-like consistency. They are extremely nutritious and ideally used in convalescence.

When To Take: To maximize absorption, herbs should be taken on an empty stomach about one hour before eating. However, if the herb causes a slight stomach upset then the tea can be taken one hour after eating or after eating some fresh ginger or drinking fresh ginger juice.

the ginseng jar on top of a small cloth or towel when in the bigger pot). Drink one cup of tea before bed and another on rising.

CHINESE LICORICE

Radix glycyrrhizae uralensis (sweet grass)

Named the "great peacemaker" by the Chinese, this soothing herb is an excellent calmer for the digestive system while also working as a mild laxative and relieving sore throats, coughing and wheezing. Because of its unique property of affecting the major meridians, it appears in many prescriptions. It is virtually universal and used in preparing preserved fruits.

Chinese Licorice Root Tea

(2 servings)

4 x 0.25cm (1-inch) pieces of Chinese licorice root

4 cups water

Honey to taste

Bring four cups of water to the boil in a saucepan. Add licorice root and simmer for 20 minutes or until liquid is reduced by half. Strain and sweeten with honey if needed.

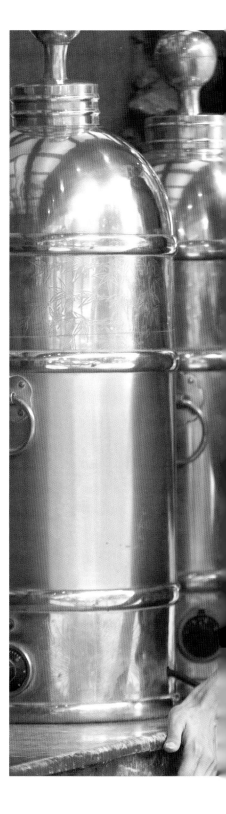

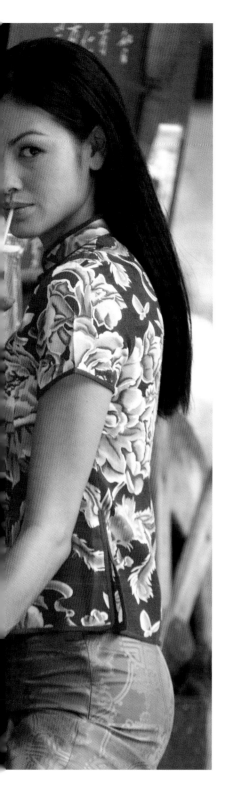

DANDELION

Herba taraxacum officinale (fisherman's herb)

An excellent spring healer, the characteristic bitterness of the dandelion's roots cleanses and stimulates all the glands involved with digestion, especially the liver. It is also used to treat mastitis, urinary infections, swollen eyes and as a lactation promoter. Dandelion greens are very nourishing and excellent in salads or drunk as a tea.

Dandelion Tonic

(1 serving)

4-5 carrots

Handful of dandelion leaves

1 fennel bulb

Lemon juice to taste

Blend all ingredients together and drink immediately.

WOLFBERRY

Semen schizandrae

These tiny sweet berries are orange to red in colour depending on the region of China in which they are grown. They are generally taken as tea or soup (both savoury and sweet) to help promote the healthy functioning of *Qi* and blood. Nourishing the blood, wolfberries are also commonly used to treat anaemia. They are excellent in the treatment of arthritis and dry skin while also promoting clear and radiant eyes.

Preparing Chinese Herbal Teas

When using Chinese herbs the following basic guidelines will ensure you get the maximum benefit from the herb. If more specific advice is needed, please consult your Chinese practitioner or herbalist.

Containers: Ceramic or glass are best. Pots or teapots must have lids to ensure no goodness is lost. Avoid cast iron or metal as they can alter the therapeutic qualities of the herbs.

Cooking: Soak herbs in water before cooking. The water should come to about 5cm (1.5 inches) above the herbs. Let this sit for 15 minutes or so before turning on the heat. Bring to the boil then reduce heat to a simmer. The average cooking time is about 20 minutes (less if using the flowers of herbs and up to 30 minutes for some tonic herbs). To maximize therapeutic effects, always keep covered. Strain the tea and drink. The same herbs can be recooked a second time. If the taste is unpalatable then water down a little. Honey may be added to some herbal teas to make them sweeter. However, it is best to check with a doctor or herbalist first as honey can adversely affect the therapeutic qualities of certain herbs.

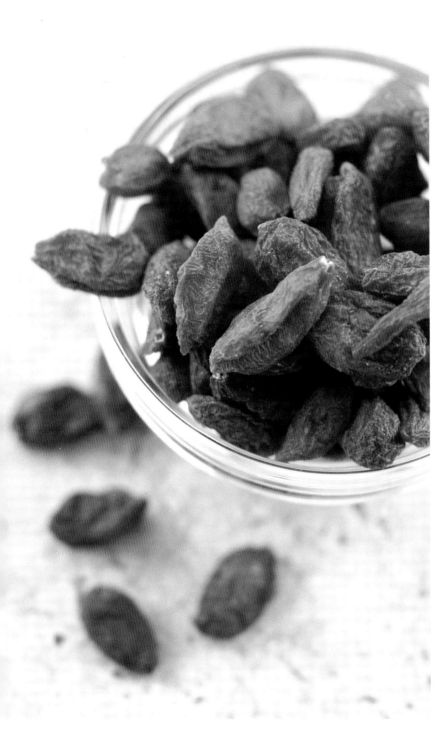

Wolfberry Tea

(*2 servings*)

2-3 tbsp dried wolfberries

2 cups water

Honey to taste

Place wolfberries and water in a saucepan and bring to the boil. Stir, cover and reduce heat. Simmer over low heat for approximately five minutes. Sweeten with honey if desired and drink immediately.

BIRD'S NEST

Collocalia inexpectata (Asian swiftlets' nests)

Bird's nest is a gastronomic delicacy. It is literally a nest created by sea swallows native to Southeast Asia. Rather than collecting twigs and debris, the birds secrete a gelatinous saliva which hardens into a nest and sticks to the walls of the caves they make home. Medicinally, bird's nest is primarily indicated in convalescence—promoting digestion and absorption and helping delay the onset of ageing. It strengthens the lungs and is used to treat chronic bronchitis and emphysema.

Stewed Bird's Nest with Almonds

(*1 serving*)

20g (0.8oz) bird's nest

40g (1.6oz) large sweet almonds (peeled)

40g (1.6oz) rock sugar

1 ½ cups water

Soak bird's nest in boiling water for about two hours. Repeat with cold water. Wash sweet almonds. Add ½ cup of water to almonds and grate them to make a fine almond juice. Strain. Put bird's nest into a stewing pot, add sugar and one cup of boiling water. Stew over high heat for 30 minutes. Serve this glutinous soup hot.

CHAMOMILE

Matricaria chamomilla

A herb for the stomach and spleen, chamomile is one of the oldest and most popular herbs. Drunk as a tea it soothes and calms the stomach. It is also excellent for menstrual problems. Used on the eyes, chamomile relieves tiredness and irritation. Simply soak cottonwool pads in cold chamomile tea and place over the eyes. Lie down and relax while the herb soothes the eyes.

Chamomile Tea

(4 servings)

2 tbsp fresh or 1 tbsp dried chamomile flowers

½ litre (1 pint) boiling water

Honey to taste

Put chamomile flowers in a teapot and pour boiling water over them. Cover and let stand for 10-15 minutes. Add honey to taste and drink.

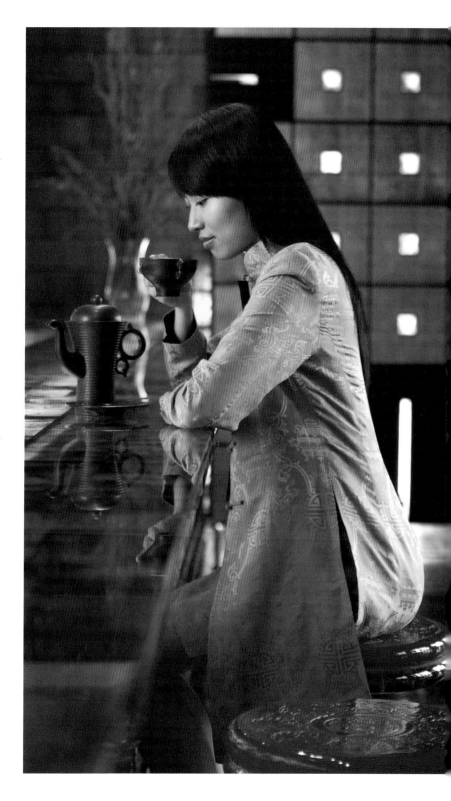

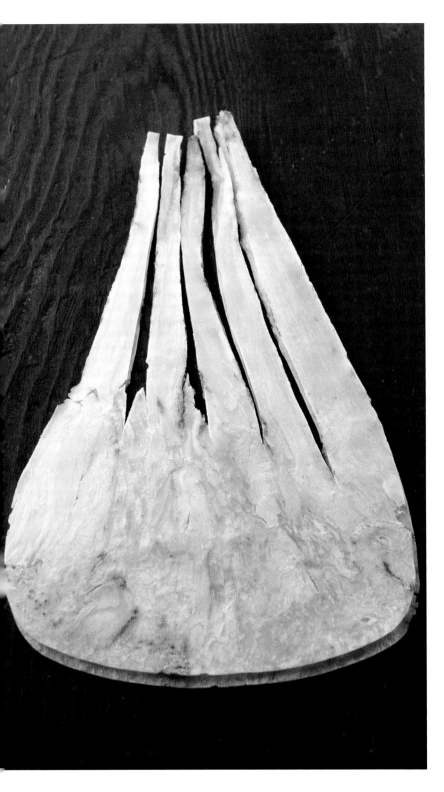

DANG GUI (OR DONG QUAI)

Radix angelica sinensis (Chinese angelica)

Considered the queen of women's herbs, *dang gui* (pictured left) is one of the most widely used herbs in China as it is beneficial to the blood, regulating the menstrual cycle and invigorating the entire system. As well as dilating the blood vessels, the herb has anti-inflammatory, analgesic and antibacterial effects and is routinely prescribed for the relief of cramps and other menstrual symptoms as well as the hot flushes associated with menopause. *Dang gui* is eaten raw or cooked, alone or combined with other herbs, in capsules or liquid form. Generally the whole root is cut into longitudinal slices and used either boiled with sweet dates (such as jujube) to make a sweet tea or in chicken or mutton soup (see below). Such a soup is said to replenish a woman's hormones if drunk three times a week.

Double-boiled Dang Gui and Chicken Soup

(*4 servings*)

12g (0.4oz) *dang gui*

1 whole chicken (cut into pieces)

Place ingredients in a non-metal pot. Place this inside another pot with 6-10cm (2-3 inches) of water. Bring to the boil and continue boiling for 2-3 hours. Put through a sieve and drink the clear soup.

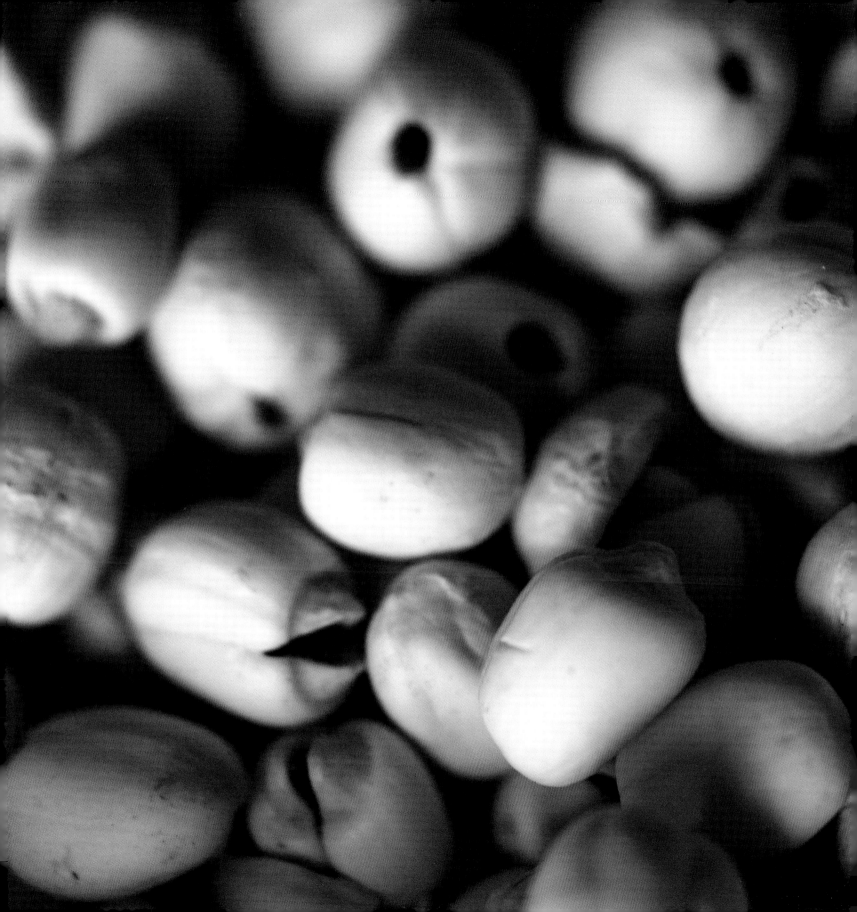

Cleanse Your Body

Is your system overloaded?

The body's primary elimination organs are the liver, kidney, skin, bowel and lymphatic system. When they become overloaded they get sluggish and less efficient, and toxic symptoms start to appear. Detoxing is the body's spring clean—cleansing the organs, clearing toxic build-up and returning balance and harmony to the entire system.

SYMPTOMS OF IMBALANCE IN THE BODY

The Liver: Bloating, nausea, indigestion and a furry tongue.

The Lungs: Runny nose, constant sneezing or sinus problems.

The Kidneys: Strong-smelling urine and a sluggish system.

The Lymphatic System: Frequent colds and flu, tiredness, cellulite and fluid retention.

The Skin and Face: Congested, blotchy, dehydrated skin, dark circles under the eyes, bad breath and a furry tongue.

The Intestine: Abdominal problems—constipation, gas and wind.

Do not perform any type of detox or liver flush if:

⊕ **You are not well or are just recovering from an illness.**

⊕ **You have gallstones or are diabetic or have any abnormalities with your blood sugar levels.**

⊕ **You are pregnant or breastfeeding.**

⊕ **You are taking any medication or being treated by your doctor for a particular complaint.**

As with any detoxing program it is advisable to first consult a Chinese medical physician who may also prescribe detox herbs and tonics.

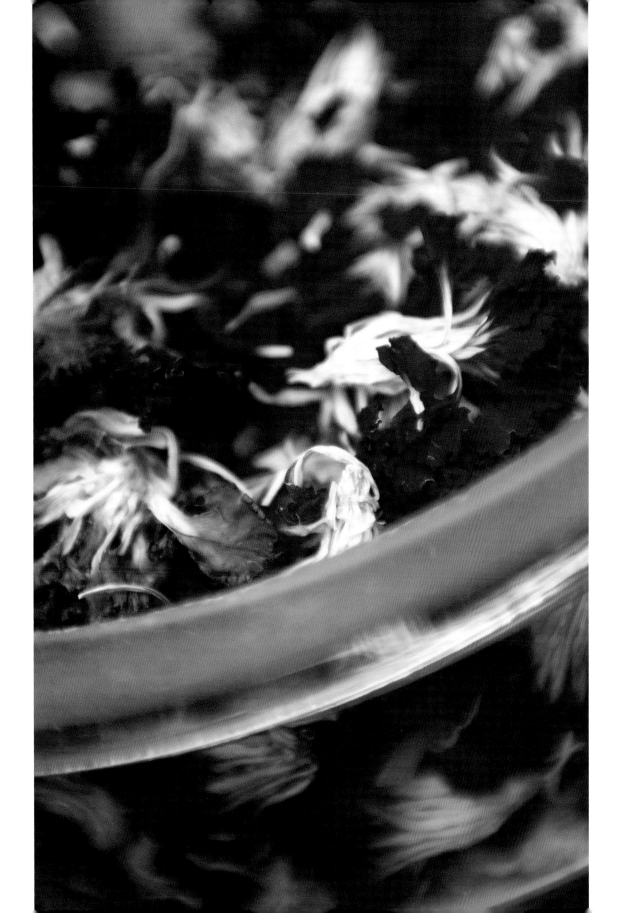

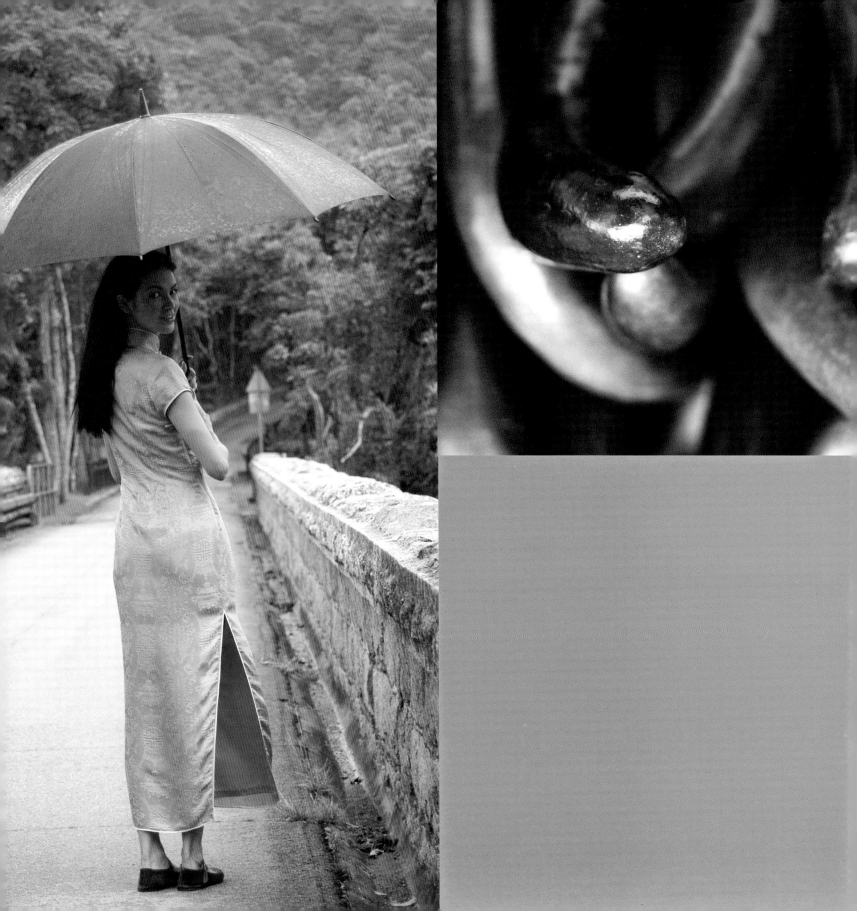

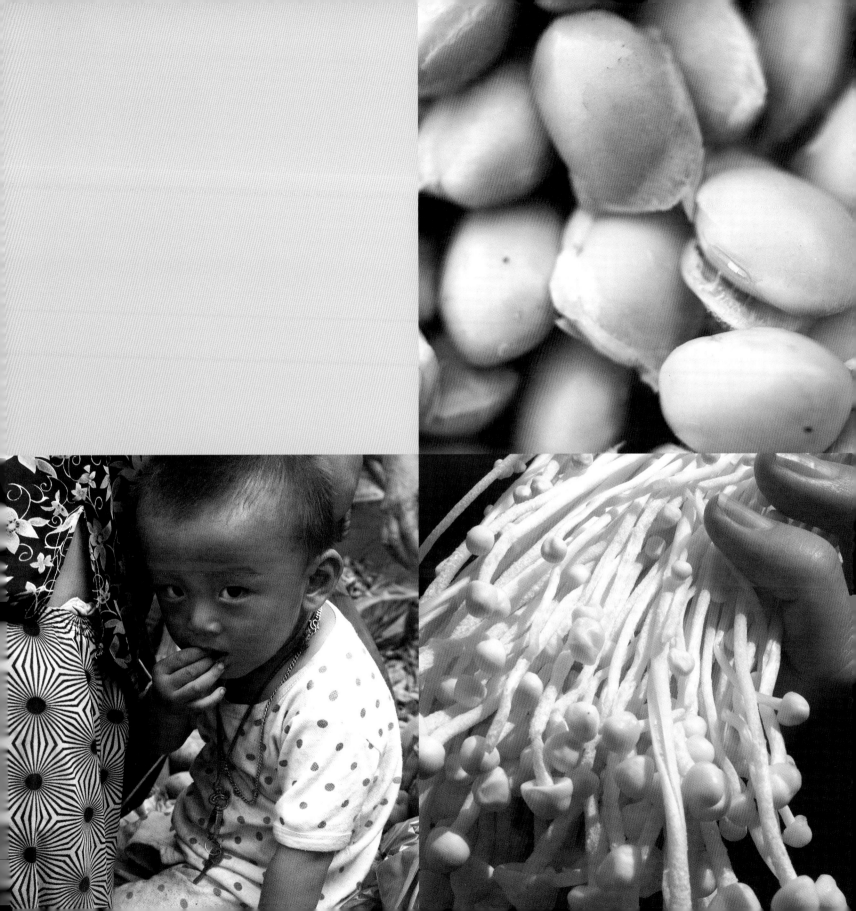

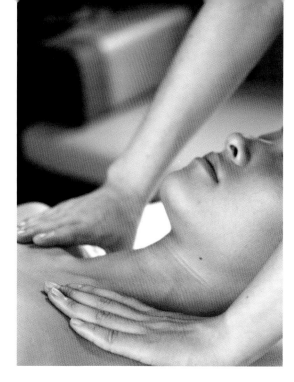
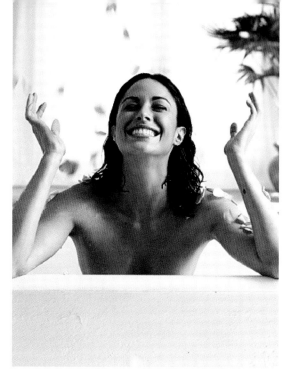

Fourteen-Day Cleanse

This is a time for you—make the most of it.

Relax. Invest in a good-quality body brush or loofah. Burn soothing and cleansing aromatherapy oils like lime, lemon, juniper, chamomile and lavender. Read, take baths, enjoy massage, listen to music or simply clear your mind. As with any successful detox, you may feel worse before you feel better which is a sure sign that the body is cleansing. The long-term results are well worth it.

FOODS TO EAT:

Fruits and nuts: lemon and lime juice, apples, pears, strawberries, cherries, blueberries, prunes, watermelon, peach, papaya, kiwifruit, walnuts.

Vegetables: carrots, yams or sweet potatoes, green beans, beetroot, squash (all types), celery, peas, onions, garlic, chives, scallions, pumpkin, cauliflower, Jerusalem artichoke, alfalfa sprouts, asparagus, turnips, beets, peppers, leeks, tomatoes, miso, brussel sprouts, chard, eggplant, okra, potatoes, parsnips, spinach and members of the cabbage family (watercress, mustard, horseradish, radish, kohlrabi, cabbage, *bak choi*, *choi sum* and kale).

Protein foods: skinless chicken and turkey, tuna, salmon (not smoked) and other fish, wild game and soya.

Grains and seeds: adzuki (red) and other bean varieties, quinoa, buckwheat, millet, barley, brown and wild rice, rice cakes, oats, sunflower seeds.

Herbs, spices and condiments: turmeric, dandelion greens, basil, bay leaf, cardamom, cumin, curry, caraway seeds, cinnamon, chives, fennel, parsley, nutmeg, rosemary, tarragon, marjoram, dill, ginger, honey, poppy seeds, herbal teas (except citrus varieties), olive oil.

Other daily essentials:

- Probiotic supplements (packed with live strains of gut-friendly bacteria to maintain intestinal balance and health; available as powder or capsules).*
- Multivitamin and mineral supplement.*
- Flaxseed oil: 1 tsp per day.
- Water: 1 ½-2 litres of warm(ish) water per day.

* Follow manufacturer's dosage instructions.

Foods to avoid:

- Meats, milk and dairy products (eggs, cream, cheese, chocolate and yoghurt).
- Foods with hydrogenated or "trans-fatty acids" such as most margarines, packaged and fast foods—check food labels.
- Coffee, alcohol, drugs (including most medications which are toxic to the liver).
- Peanuts and coconut products (although young coconut milk is accepted).
- Spicy foods (as they can upset the liver).

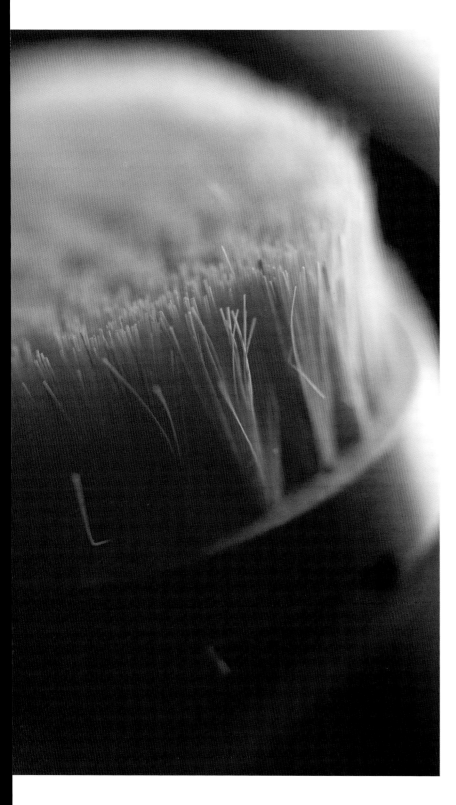

Days 1-3:
Initial Unloading Phase

On rising:

A cup of warm water with a squeeze of lemon or lime juice

    (a touch of honey can be added if desired)

Dry body brush before showering (see pages 87 and 97)

Breakfast

Fruit (fresh, juiced, stewed or poached)

    or detox juices (page 80)

Mid Morning

Fruit and herbal tea (ginseng or Chinese licorice, pages 61 and 64)

Lunch and Dinner

Only meals prepared from "Foods to Eat" list (pages 74-75)

Days 4-7:
Cleansing Phase

On rising:

A cup of warm water with a squeeze of lemon or lime juice

    (a touch of honey can be added if desired)

Epsom salts (1 tbsp mixed with a large glass of warm water)

Dry body brush before showering

Breakfast

Liver detox cereal (page 81) mixed with 1 tsp
    flaxseed oil

Mid Morning

$^1\!/_2$ papaya or 2 kiwifruit plus one pear or a slice
    watermelon

Lunch

Vegetable soup (page 81)

Mid Afternoon

Fresh fruit or vegetable juice

Dinner

Same as breakfast or a large bowl of vegetable soup

Day 8-9:
The Liver Flush

(see page 79)

Day 10-14:
Rebuilding Phase

Same as Days 1-3 (Initial Unloading Phase)

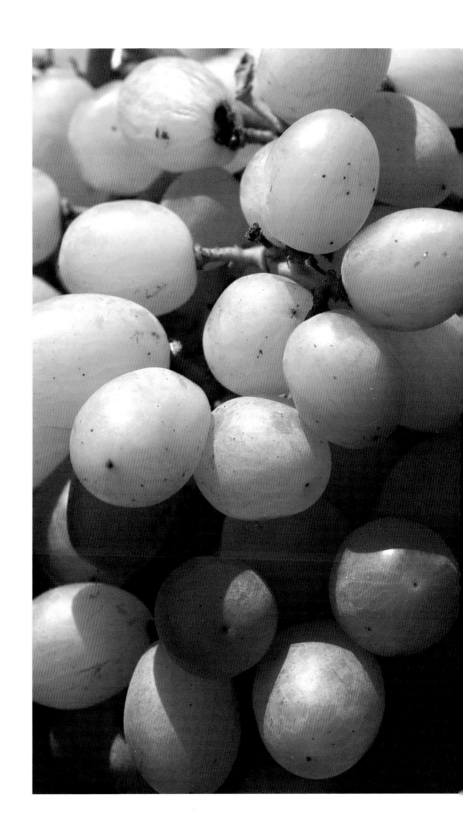

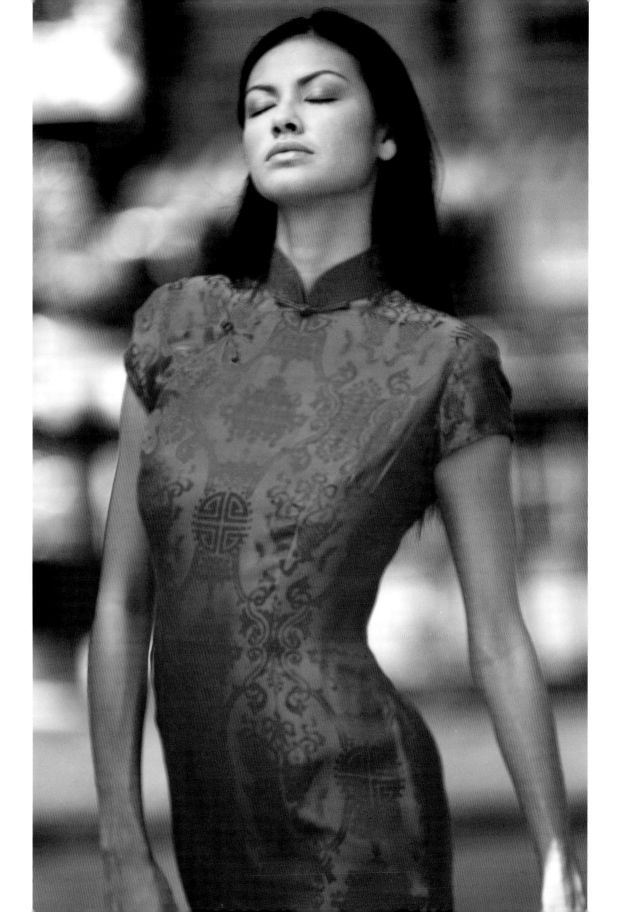

THE LIVER FLUSH

The liver flush clears stagnation in the liver and is ideally carried out at the end of the first week of cleansing. It can also be repeated to coincide with seasonal change, after periods of excess or to further weight loss but should not be carried out more than four times per year. Flushing is best done over a weekend or when you have a complete rest day as you will need to stay close to a bathroom. Please consult a physician (Western or Chinese) before conducting the liver flush.

You will need:

1 bottle virgin olive oil

6 lemons

60g (2.4oz) Epsom Salts

3 litres water

Day 1:

To prepare for the Liver Flush take fruit juices or soup for breakfast and lunch on the first day. Drink at least 1 1/2 litres of water during the afternoon before doing the following:

6.30pm: Drink 1 heaped tbsp Epsom salts mixed into a large glass of warm water

7.30pm: Same as 6.30pm followed by a few mouthfuls of water to rinse. Shower and dry then body brush in a upward motion towards the heart

8.30pm: Squeeze six lemons to get about 100ml pure lemon juice. Add this to 200ml of olive oil (at room temperature) and blend together. Over the following 1 $\frac{1}{2}$ hours drink this mixture (about a quarter at a time) until finished. When in bed do not lie on the right side to keep the liver clear

DAY 2:

6.30am: Drink 1 heaped tbsp Epsom salts mixed into a large glass of warm water. You can start to eat light food after 8.00am but do not stray far from the bathroom.

Fourteen-Day Cleansing Recipes

DETOX JUICES

Daily juicing is essential. Fruits and vegetables share profound healing properties and encourage elimination. The alkaline nature of vegetables helps bind acids and eliminate them via the kidneys and urine.

- ❖ **Carrot juice**: Improves digestion and an excellent source of the powerful antioxidant vitamin A.
- ❖ **Dandelion tonic**: page 65.
- ❖ **Beetroot juice**: Enriches the blood and an excellent tonic for the kidneys.
- ❖ **Celery juice**: On its own or juiced with apple this makes a deliciously refreshing and cleansing drink.
- ❖ **Cleansing liver tonic**: A powerful blend of one beetroot, two carrots and two to three celery sticks with the added sweetness of the juice of one orange.
- ❖ **Fruit juice blend**: Blend the following fruits together: kiwi, mango, papaya, pears, persimmons, red apples, red grapefruit, 1 cup red grapes, 1 cup strawberries, tangerine, watermelon (with 1 cup of white rind).

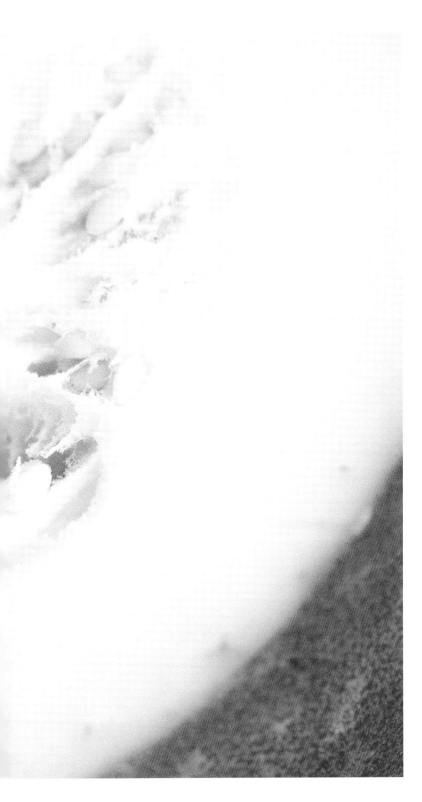

Liver Detox Cereal

(*2 servings*)

$^1/_2$ piece dried fungus

$^1/_2$ cup dried chestnuts, chopped

$^1/_2$ cup dried red dates

$^1/_4$ cup lily bulb (choose white variety)

$^1/_4$ cup pearl barley

$^1/_2$ cup dried lotus seed (soaked in water for 8 hours)

$^1/_2$ cup lycium berries

Honey or rock sugar to taste

Taken as a soup, this is best prepared the night before. Mix all ingredients together and place in an earthenware pot with 600ml water. Bring to the boil and simmer for 30 minutes until the barley is soft.

Vegetable Soup

(*4 servings*)

2 large unpeeled but clean potatoes, sliced

I cup carrots, finely chopped

I cup beetroot, finely chopped

I cup fresh beans, finely chopped

I cup celery, finely chopped

I cup one other vegetable (cabbage, watercress, horseradish, broccoli, kohlrabi, *bak choi* or kale), finely chopped

Put ingredients in a large pot, cover with 2 litres of water. Cook for 30 minutes, cool, strain and serve. Keep in refrigerator and warm when needed.

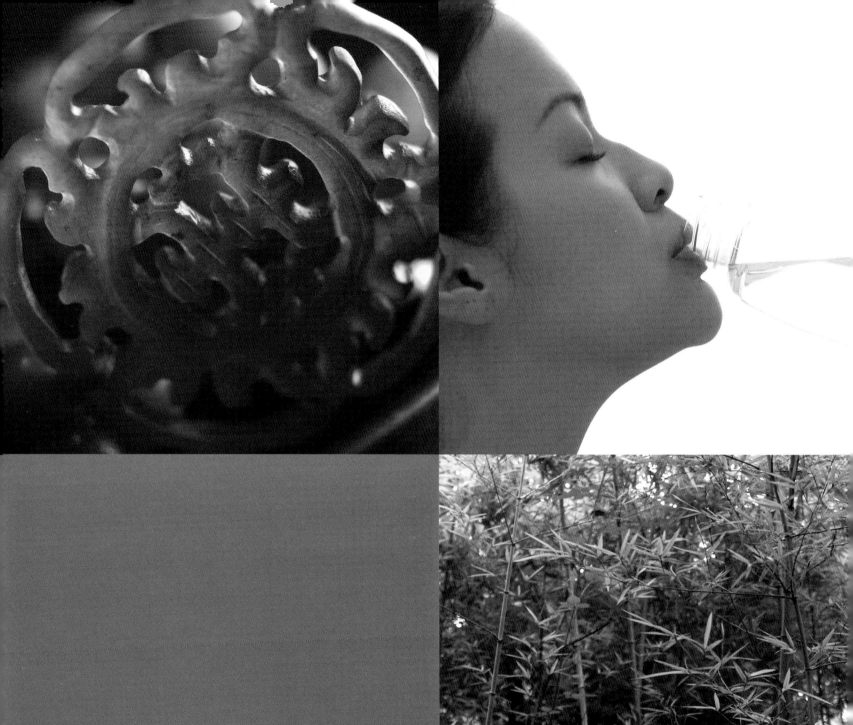

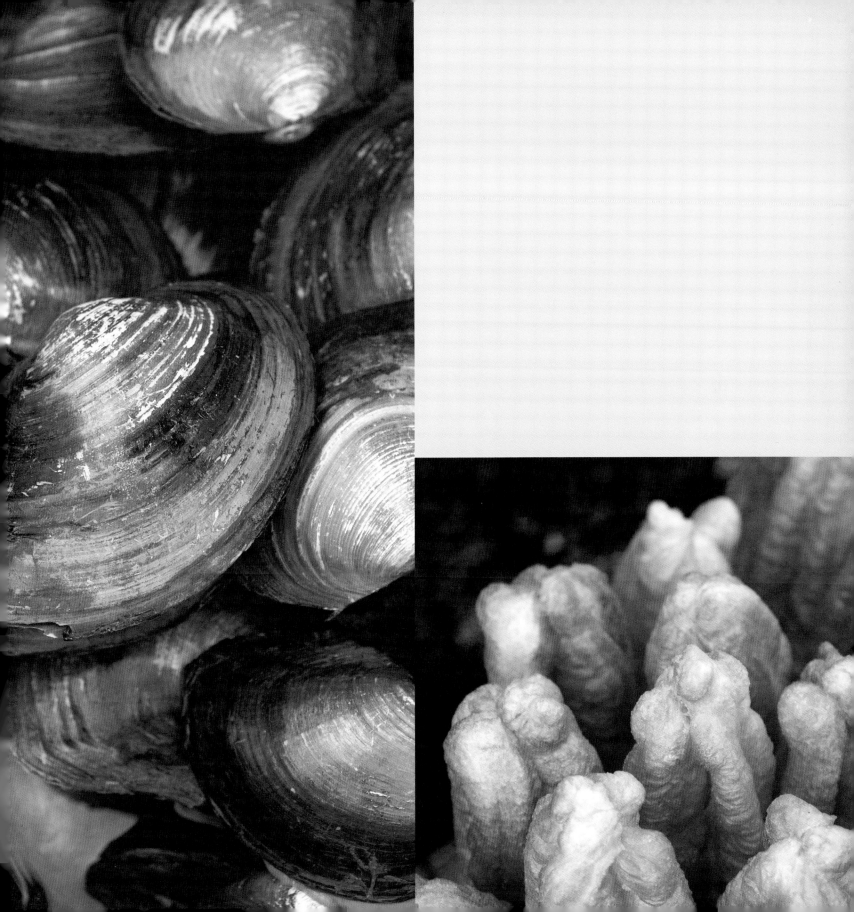

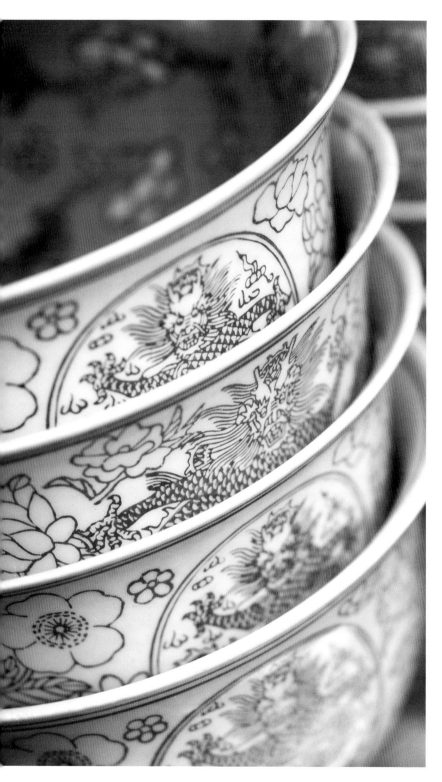

CLEANSING TEAS

Ginseng Tea: page 61.

Chinese Licorice Root Tea: page 64.

Chrysanthemum Tea

(1 serving)

1 tbsp chrysanthemum flowers

1 cup boiling water

Infuse chrysanthemum flowers in a cup of boiling water.
Allow to steep. Drink either hot or cold.

Wild Orchid Tea

(2 servings)

$^1/_2$ cup dried Chinese orchids *(Herba dendrobii* or *suk gok)*

1 slice Chinese licorice root,
     about 1.25cm (0.5 inch) long

4 cups water

Honey to taste

Bring water to the boil. Add herbs and reduce heat to
simmer for 20 minutes or until liquid is reduced by half.
Strain off herbs and sweeten with honey if desired.
Drink warm.

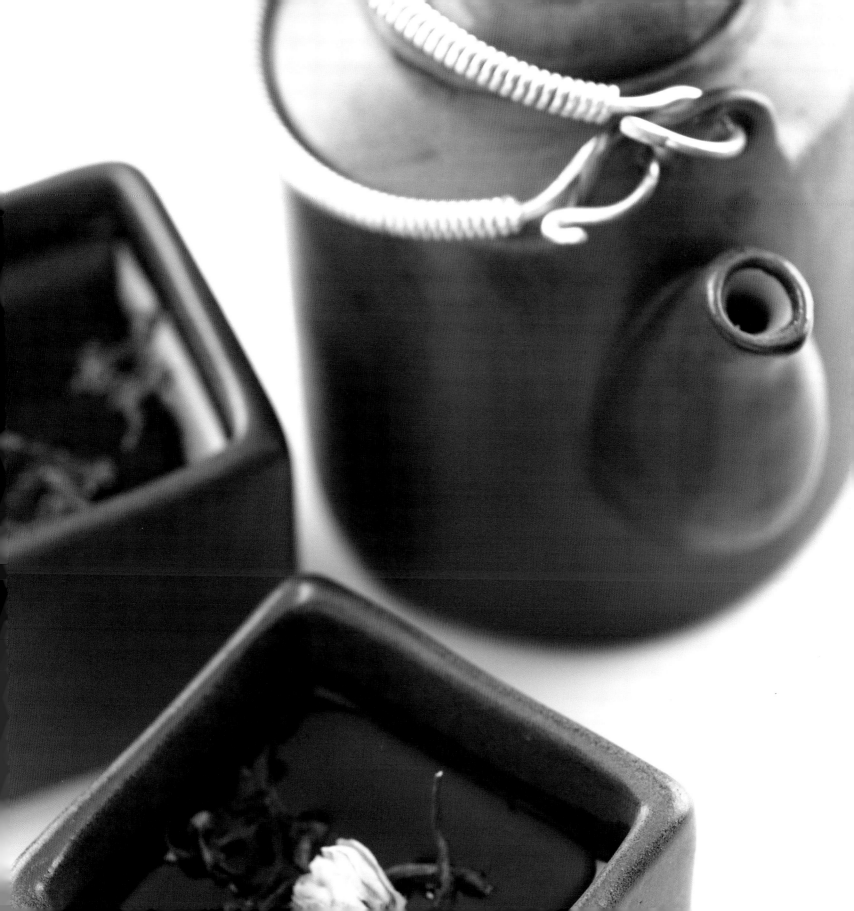

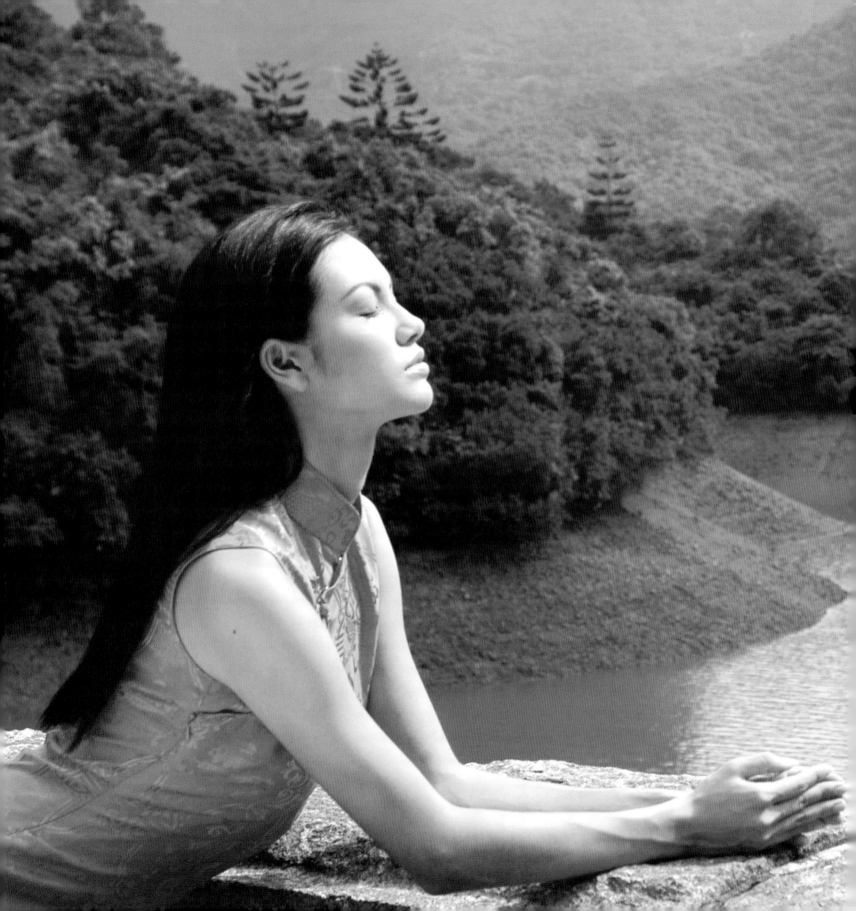

Detoxing Extras

BODY BRUSHING

This gentle yet powerful technique breaks down congestion in stagnant body parts by stimulating internal movement and draining the lymphatic system. Just five minutes in the morning before showering (always brushing towards the heart) can make a big difference (see also page 97).

SAUNAS

Dry saunas promote sweating and the release of fat-soluble toxins through the skin. It is recommended to stay in the sauna for a minimum of 30 minutes (inclusive of short breaks) so the temperature must not be excessive. Shower well afterwards to ensure toxins are completely removed. Take flaxseed oil daily to replace lost essential fats.

Don't expect to look completely different after just 14 days—but you will feel lighter, brighter, energized and more alive.

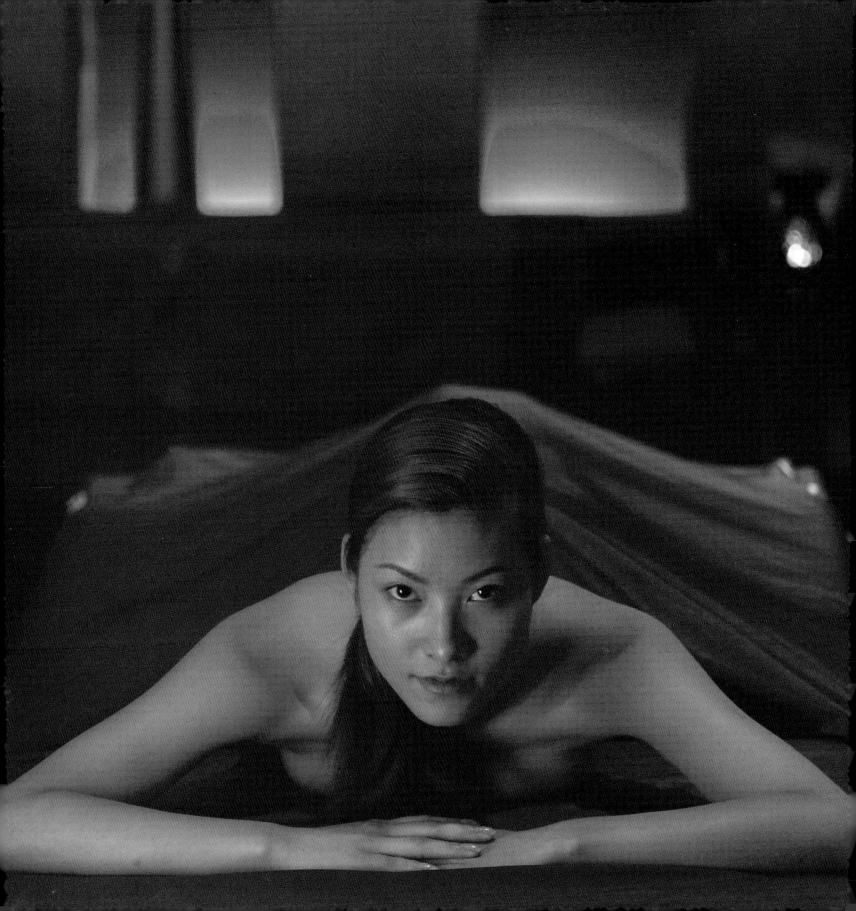

CHAPTER 3

Chinese Spa and Movement Therapies:

massage, qi gung and tai chi

"Flowing water never stagnates. The hinges of an active door never rust. This is due to movement. The same principle applies to essence and energy. If the body does not move, *Qi* does not flow and energy stagnates."

— *Spring and Autumn Annals* (4th Century BC)

Spa Therapies

Massage is believed to have originated in the East as a method of unblocking *Qi*. It heals and helps the skin. Kneading, stroking or pressing helps clear energy channels, release tension and create more body-mind-emotion harmony.

The Chinese massage practitioner must have a thorough understanding of the principles of medicine to make a diagnosis and practise specific hands-on techniques. Depending on the particular situation one or a combination of the following massage techniques will be used to restore balance and control to the body.

ACUPRESSURE

Acupressure is a term encompassing any number of massage techniques that use manual pressure to stimulate energy points in the face and body. "Acu" means care or precision and the acupressure system of therapy shares the same points on the body as does acupuncture. However, instead of using needles, the therapist uses hands and fingers to stimulate acupoints and enhance circulation through the meridians.

For example, a simple acupressure technique for eye strain and headache is to gently massage the acupressure points on both sides of the ridge of the nose, next to the eyes, to move *Qi* and ease the discomfort. By keeping the face nourished through a continuously circulating supply of *Qi* and blood, acupressure facial therapy helps delay the onset of fine lines and wrinkles.

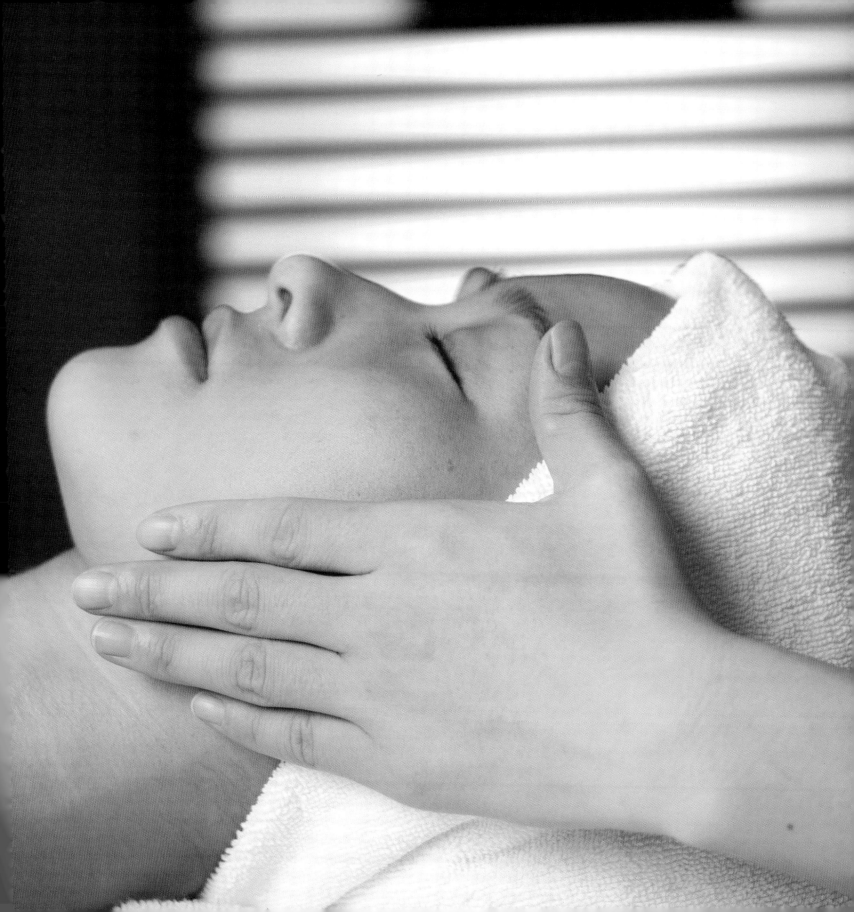

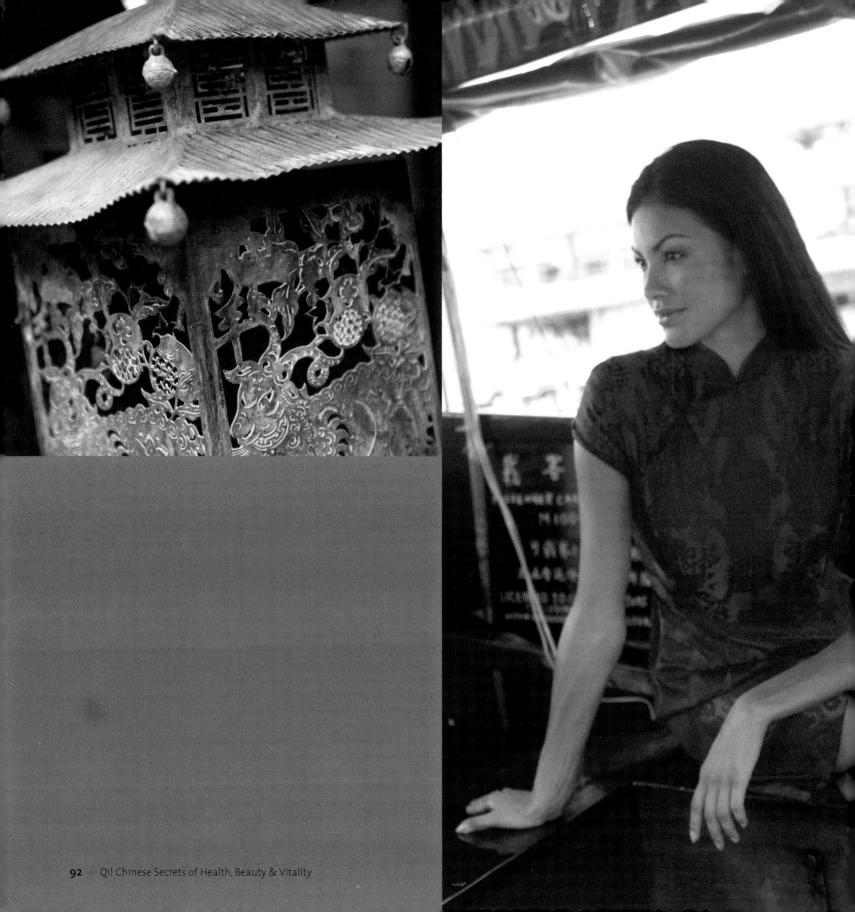

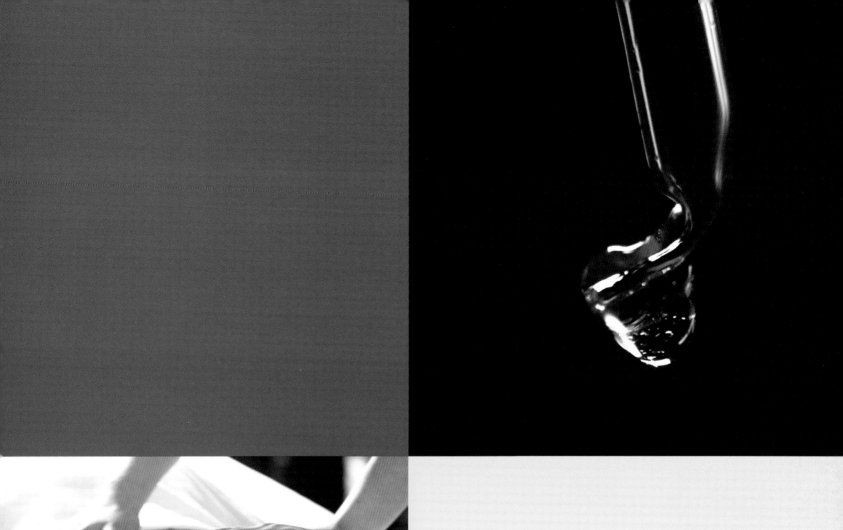
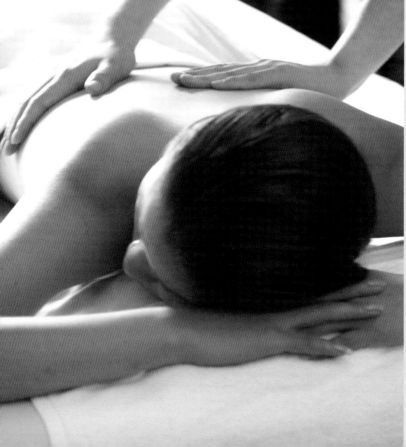

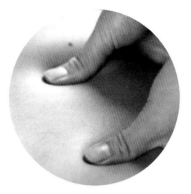

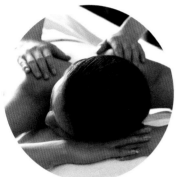

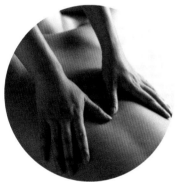

TUI NA

Literally translated as "press and rub", *tui na* is the oldest and most common form of Chinese acupressure massage. Practised for more than 4,000 years, *tui na* has won converts in western celebrities including Bruce Willis, Demi Moore, Liam Neeson, Paul McCartney and Ben Affleck. It uses deep digital stimulation to vital points along the meridians to relieve pain and fatigue, improve circulation, tone muscles and restore overall balance in the body. It is routinely used to treat a range of ailments from common colds and headaches to insomnia, intestinal upsets, menstrual irregularities, lower back pain and neck stiffness.

There are more than 20 different *tui na* techniques and the practitioner must have a thorough understanding of the principles of each to practise effectively. For example, *tui fa* (pushing technique) is used to warm the meridians and relieve pain, while *mo fa* ("round rubbing" technique) applied to the chest, stomach and head moves stagnant liver *Qi*, improving digestion and relieving headaches, insomnia and other stress-related problems.

As with other forms of massage, oils generally act as lubricants but specific preparations can also be used to treat certain ailments. For example, ginger warms the stomach and spleen and is used to treat colds, vomiting and stomach pain (see ginger and spring onion tincture, page 97) and whiskey or rice wine (used as a base for Chinese herbal tinctures) helps stimulate *Qi* and blood circulation.

REFLEXOLOGY

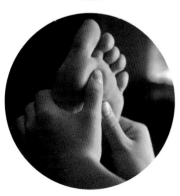

Reflexology is an ancient Chinese holistic treatment which uses pressure applied to reflex points in the feet to relieve stress and tension and improve circulation.

Six major energy meridians terminate in the feet: that of the spleen, kidneys, liver, stomach, gallbladder and bladder—as do some of the major nerves. A skilled reflexologist uses their thumbs to press and deeply massage each of the tiny reflex zones in the feet to stimulate the associated organs and glands, thereby activating the body's natural healing

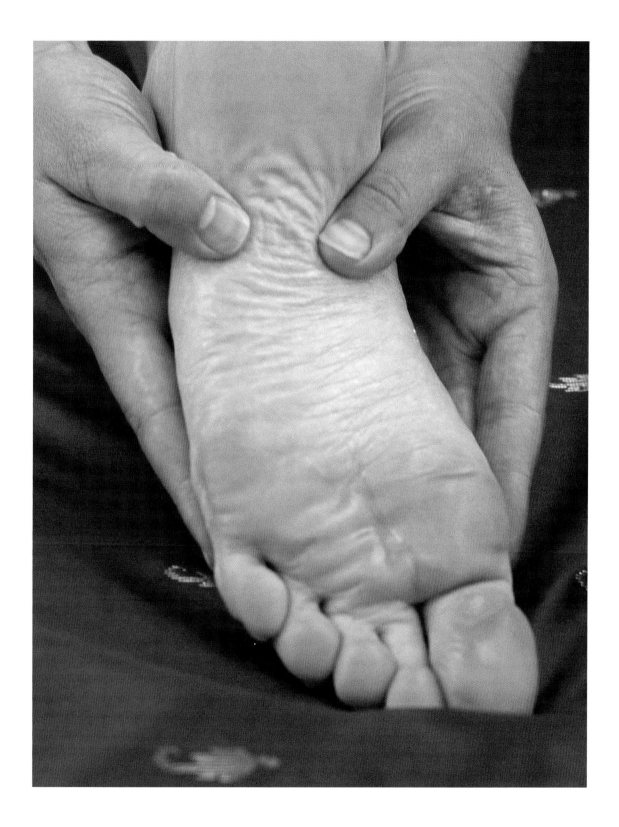

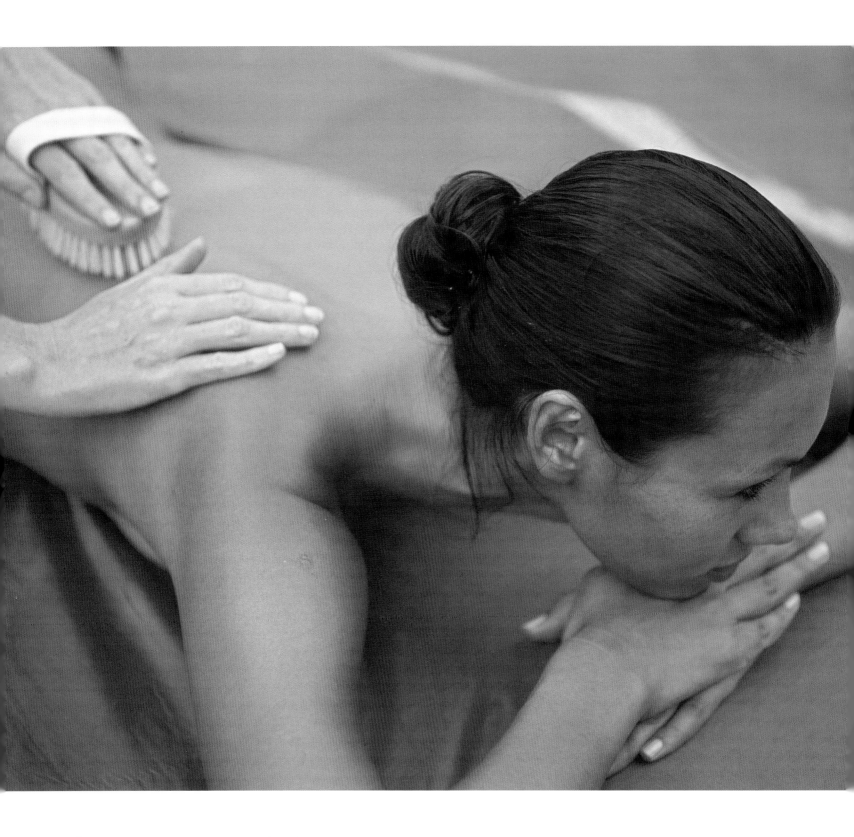

mechanisms. The heel of the foot represents the pelvic area, the bottom of the big toes links to the hormone-controlling pituitary gland and the internal organs are connected to the middle of the sole.

Reflexology has been shown to relieve a range of diseases from postnatal depression to skin conditions and the patient will often experience a sharp but short-lived pain when the zone associated with a particular imbalance is being massaged.

FIVE ELEMENT SHIATSU

Often described as acupuncture without the needles, shiatsu is a Japanese therapy that uses the application of gently applied deep finger (and sometimes palm, knuckle and elbow) pressure to remove blocked energy and rebalance the system. While based on this technique, Five Element Shiatsu goes one step further by combining shiatsu with the physical and emotional energies of the Five Elements to enhance the flow of energy through the body. It is used to relieve chronic conditions including back pain, insomnia, migraines, digestive problems, asthma or simply for pure unadulterated relaxation.

BODY BRUSHING

One of the best ways of cleansing the entire lymphatic system is to brush the surface of the body with a long-handled, soft dry brush or loofah. Once a day, preferably first thing in the morning (before showering), this simple and highly effective technique takes just a few minutes and stimulates the lymph canals to drain toxic matter into the colon, thereby purifying the system.

For best results, dry-brush the entire body (except the face) once or twice with long sweeping strokes across the skin—always towards the heart. Brush up the arms from the hands to the shoulders; up the legs from the feet to the hips; up the buttocks; down the neck and across the shoulders.

Ginger and Spring Onion Tincture
Disperses cold from the abdomen; ideal for treating colds

30g/1.2oz fresh ginger
30g/1.2oz spring onions
250ml/10 fl oz white alcohol
    (vodka or white rum)

For best results soak the ginger and spring onion in alcohol for two weeks. Strain and store. Alternatively, simmer the ginger and spring onion in water for 15 minutes and allow to cool before massaging on the abdomen.

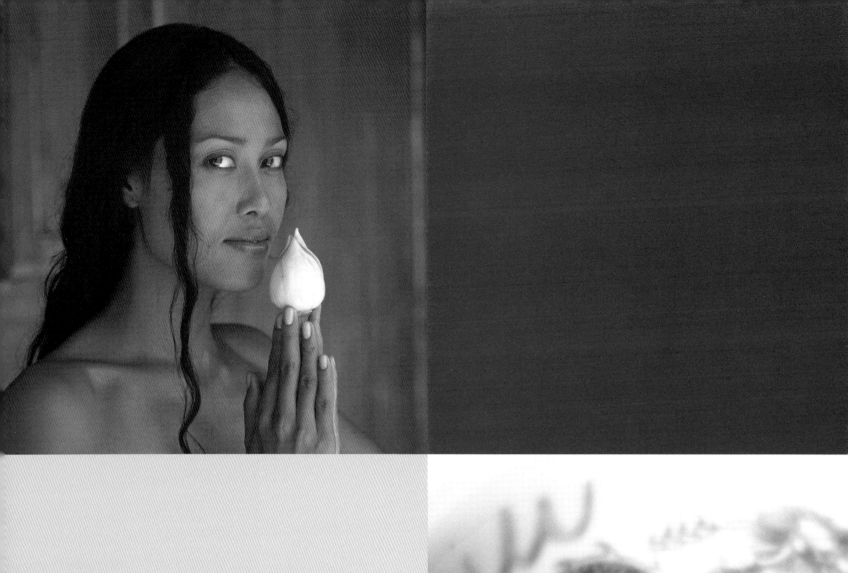
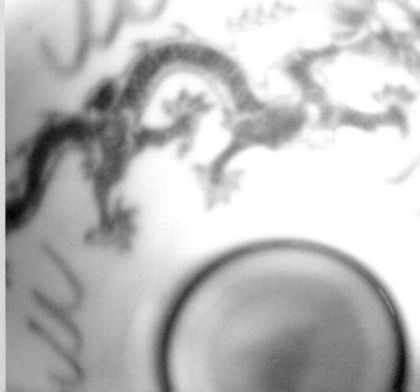

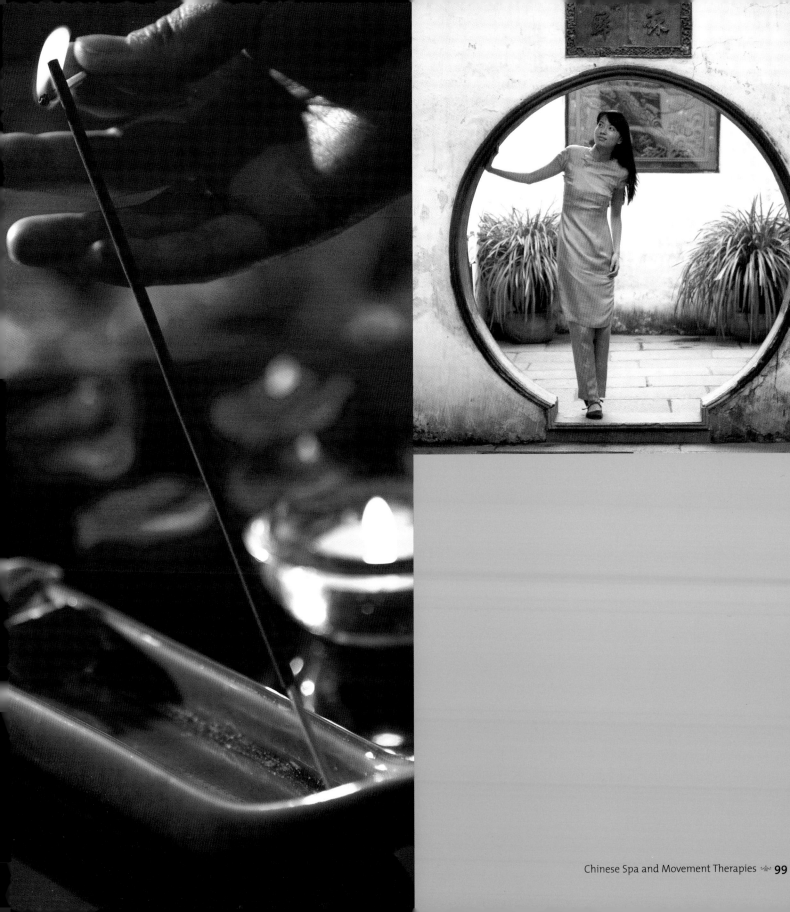

For thorough cleansing (in conjunction with the Fourteen-Day Cleanse on page 74), body brushing must be performed daily for up to three months; thereafter about twice a week. Do not scrub or rotate the brush—use long and smooth strokes to sweep across the skin.

Rinse the brush in warm water after use to clear accumulated dead skin cells. Every few weeks thoroughly clean the brush by washing it in water with a few drops of disinfecting tea-tree oil.

Movement Therapies

Soft, flowing Eastern exercises like *qi gung, tai chi* and yoga, which mirror the movement of nature, are as much a part of Chinese culture as yin and yang and the Five Elements. Far more subtle than most Western sports, they arguably offer a more powerful mind-body workout.

Each of us has our own unique exercise rhythm and with Chinese movement therapies, it is never too late to start. Central to effective practice is that the movements are soft and smooth and performed in conjunction with deep breathing. This switches the nervous system over from the chronically overactive sympathetic mode to the calming, restorative parasympathetic mode in which the body's vital functions and energies are balanced and the secretions of vital essences (like hormones) are stimulated. For this changeover to occur, the exercises must be performed slowly and with a calm mind. The equilibrium of body, mind and spirit achieved through these exercises counteracts the stresses and strains of daily life.

Qi gung, tai chi and yoga classes are widely available. To ensure you get the best start, it is advisable to contact registered societies in your area for a complete listing of qualified teachers.

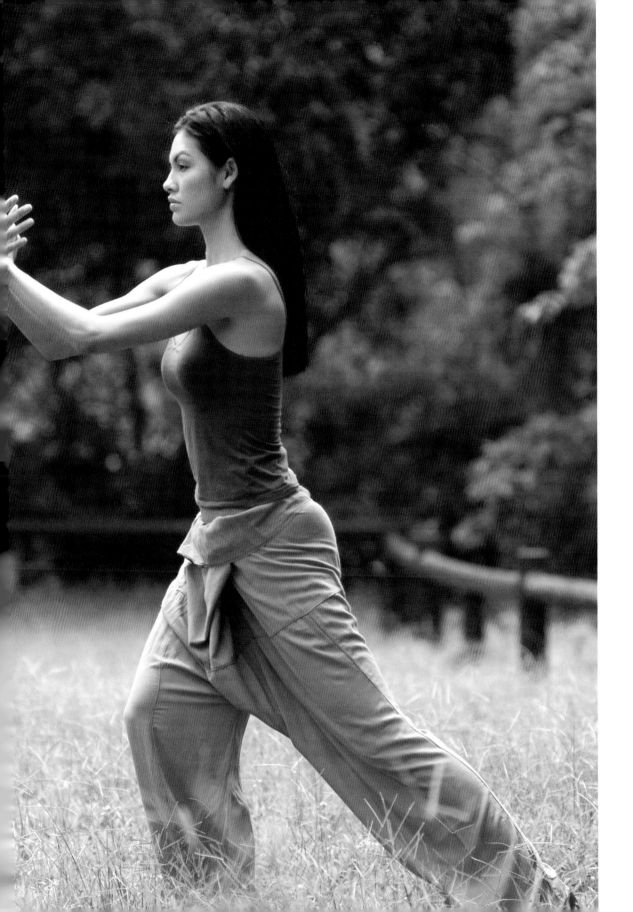

QI GUNG

First mentioned in the earliest written records of Chinese history, *qi gung* later developed into a complete system of human energy management and the most effective guardian and regulator of *Qi*.

Based primarily on movements learned by observing animals in nature, the movements were originally practised as a form of therapeutic dance to cure rheumatism and ward off other symptoms of "excess damp". With the current rebirth of Chinese philosophy, this powerful self-healing discipline has won new converts internationally.

The literal translation of *qi gung* is "energy work". These flowing, instinctive movements orchestrate balance and harmony between yin and yang, the Five Elements, the Three Treasures, and the body, brain and electromagnetic forces of our internal and external environments.

Since "blood follows where energy leads", promoting the circulation of energy through the meridians automatically enhances blood circulation through the veins, arteries and capillaries. This nourishes and energizes the organs and glands and cleanses the system of toxins and metabolic waste.

Routinely prescribed across China for the relief of chronic pain, *qi gung* is also believed to strengthen the body's resistance to disease, lower blood pressure, harmonize internal body functions, improve posture and muscle tone and, most importantly, bring body and mind to a state of peace. By increasing flexibility, stamina, balance and grace, the *qi gung* practitioner is able to gain more control of their own life force.

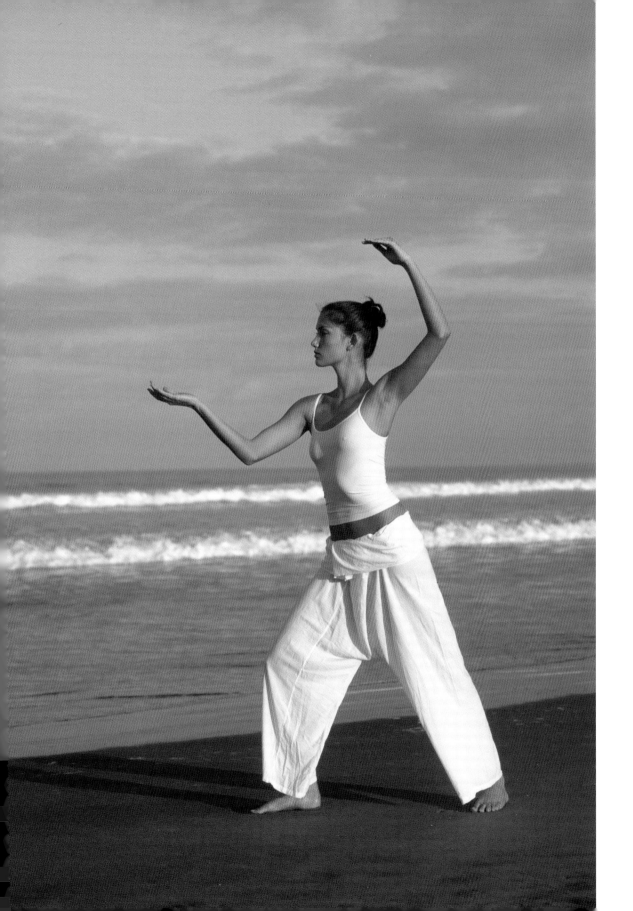

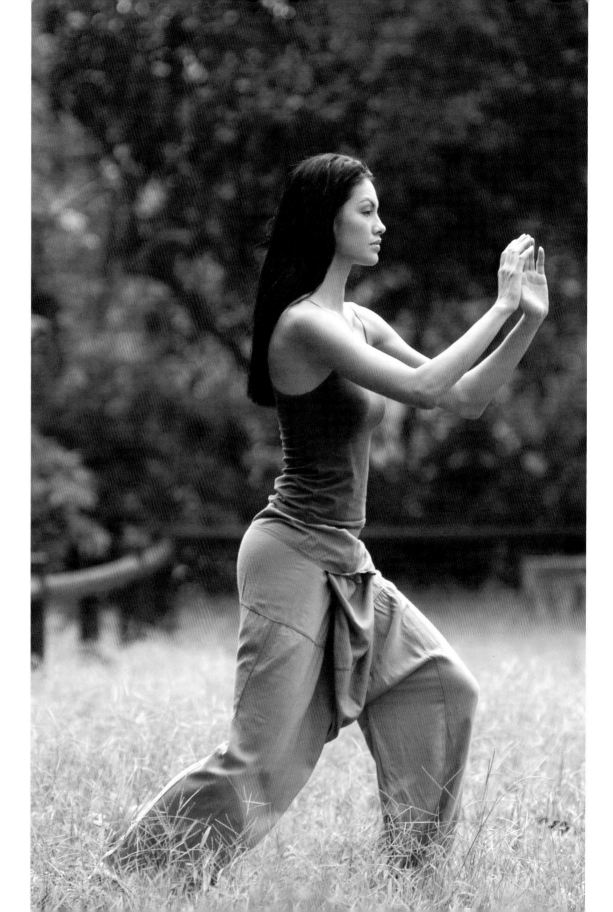

TAI CHI CHUAN

In *Tai Chi—A Way of Centering* (Collier Books, 1976), *tai chi chuan* (*tai chi* for short) is defined as "meditation in movement, a philosophical system, a set of principles of self-defense, a prophylaxis against disease, and exquisite dance. It corrects your posture and enhances relaxation. It energizes your body and tranquilizes your spirit. It is a bridge between Eastern meditation and Western psychotherapy, integrating the mind and the senses."

Literally translated as "supreme ultimate reality", *tai chi* developed out of the practice of *qi gung* by blending the internal meditation associated with *qi gung* with external exercise to further promote inner relaxation and strength. With *tai chi,* stamina and strength are developed along with grace and flexibility.

Tai chi is calming to watch and replenishing to do; many Chinese practise it in the park on their way to work.

YOGA

With its roots firmly grounded in India, yoga has proved itself far more than a hangover from the hippie Seventies. A Sanskrit word meaning "union" or "joining together", this multilevel discipline ranges from the simple daily practice of a a series of exercises called *asanas* to a complete philosophy of life incorporating diet, movement and meditation which integrates mind, body and spirit.

With regular practice yoga stimulates *Qi* and enhances the body's innate healing properties, reawakening the great power within and bringing a real feeling of peace and calm to both body and mind.

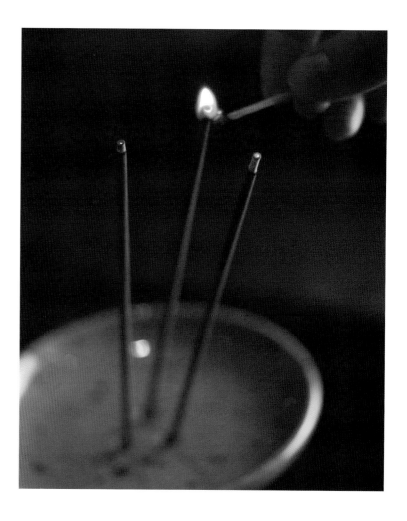

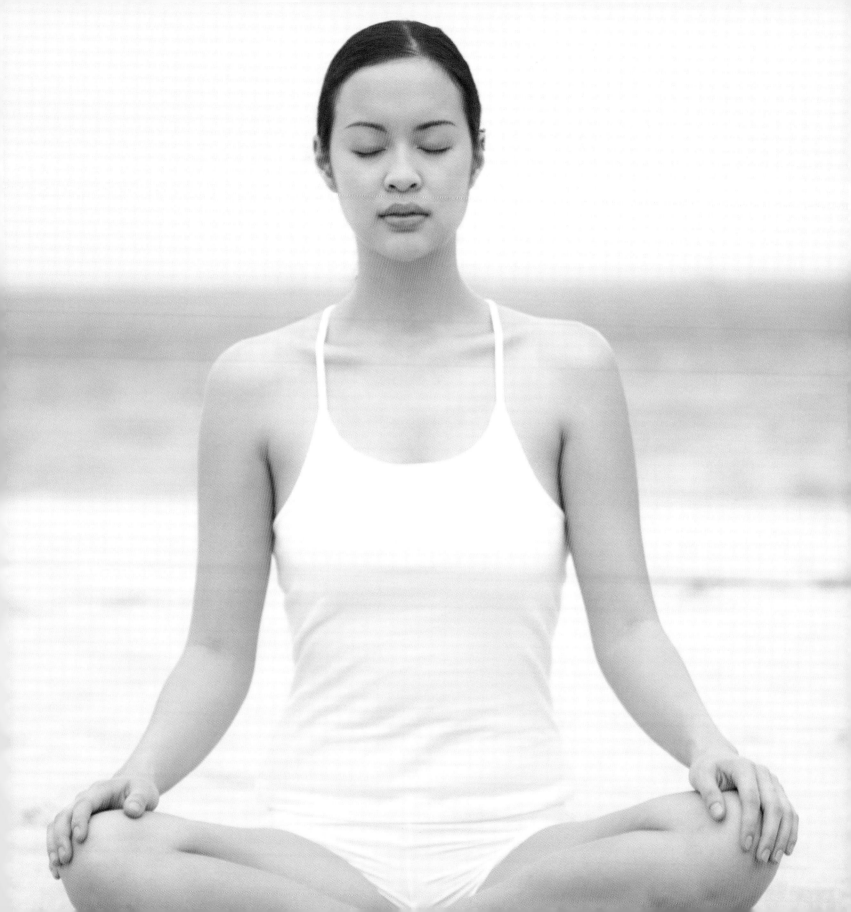

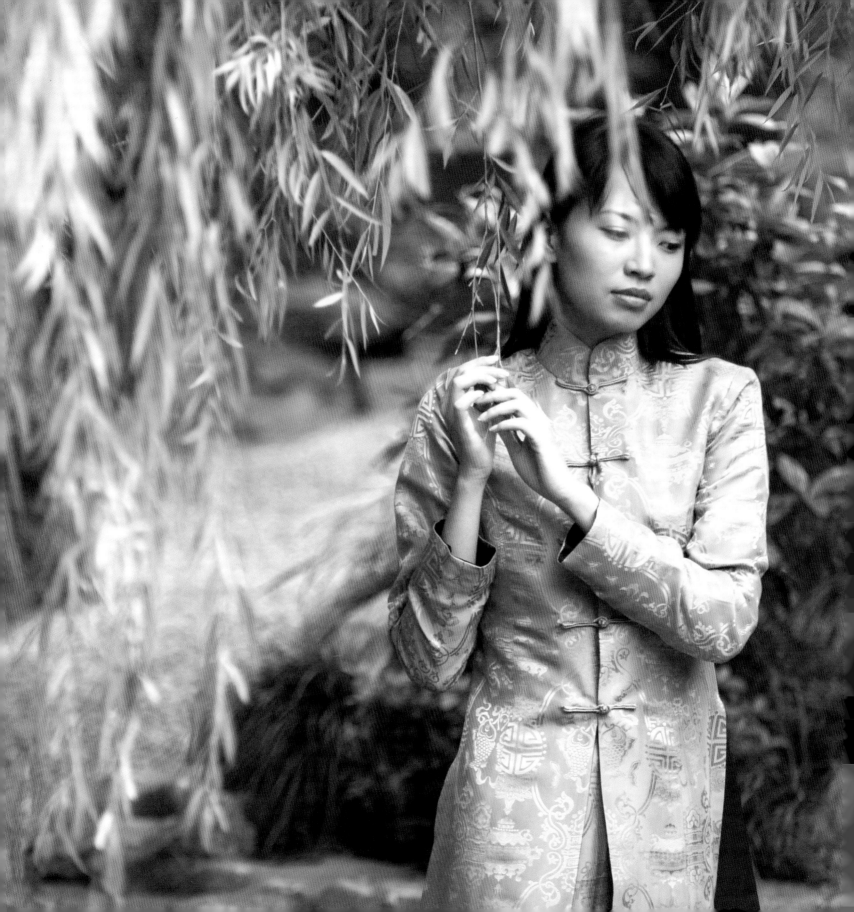

CHAPTER 4

Women's Health, Chinese-style:

menstruation, fertility and menopause

"Opening and closing the gates of heaven,
Can you play the role of woman?
Giving birth and nourishing,
Bearing yet not possessing,
Working yet not taking credit,
Leading yet not dominating,
This is the Primal Virtue."

—Lao Tzu, *Tao Te Ching* (c.1066-770BC)

The Female Cycle

In accordance with the cyclic nature of Chinese medicine, a woman's physical journey to adulthood follows a seven-year cycle, based on the movement of blood and *Qi*. At about seven years of age, blood moves to the upper part of the body and teeth mature; by about 14, refinement of blood to the uterus occurs and menstruation begins; kidney *Qi* refinement takes place at about 28 years when women are at their most fertile; and by 49 years blood starts to degenerate, the uterus becomes less functional and menopause begins.

As with these developmental stages in life, a woman's monthly cycle revolves around a series of four continuous phases starting with the first day of a period, through post-menstruation, ovulation and pre-menstruation.

Many women believe that premenstrual tension or PMT is something they have to live with every month. Not so. By simple intervention through food, herbs, exercise and, where necessary, acupuncture, most women can, and should, have a smooth and pain-free cycle. Like the nurturing relationships of the Five Elements, working with each stage of the cycle ensures a smoother transition to the next. For example, acupuncture during ovulation greatly reduces the symptoms of PMT.

For a man, *Qi* peaks at 16 and follows an eight-year cycle until the eighth cycle (i.e. 64 years) when kidney essence declines.

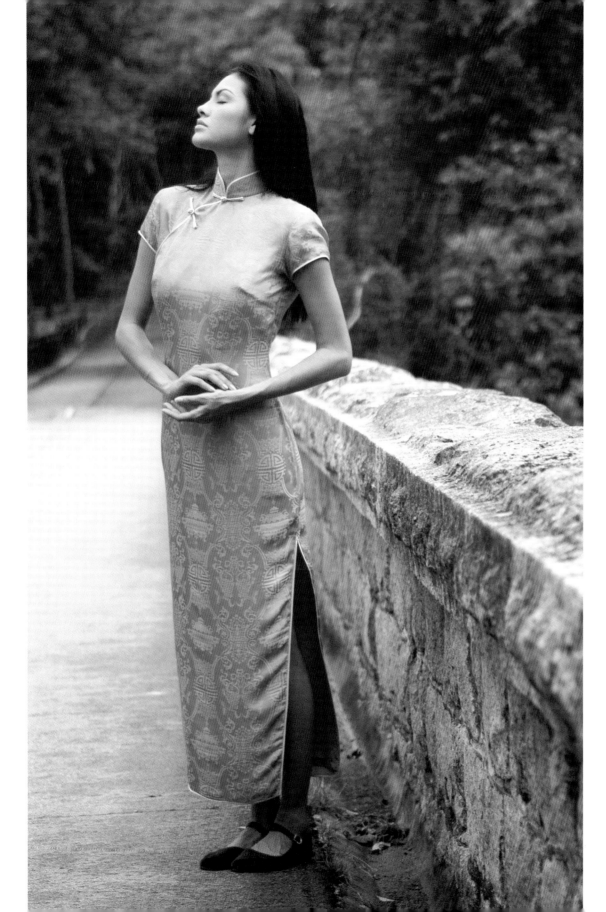

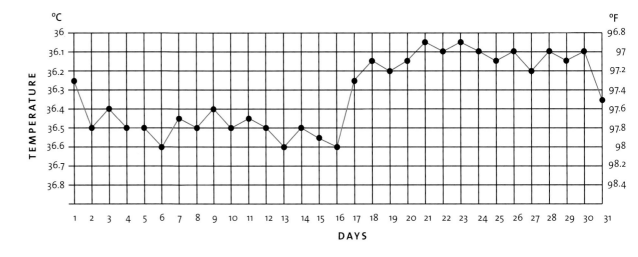

Average Daily Basal Body Temperature Over One Month

Basal Body Temperature (BBT; sometimes called the waking temperature) ideally should be taken daily at about the same time as soon as you wake after at least three hours of restful sleep. To correctly gauge the subtle but distinct difference between temperatures before and after ovulation, basal thermometers are recommended. These thermometers reach 38°C (100°F) and measure one-tenth of a degree. BBT can be affected by things such as a heated water bed or an electric blanket, alcohol consumption the night before, restless sleep, or sleeping embraced with a partner or child. Daily recording of the BBT is necessary to confirm that ovulation has taken place and the woman is at her most fertile. Ovulation generally happens within a 24-hour window before or after the temperature rise.

For those planning to become pregnant, the woman's egg must be open to penetration by the man's sperm for new life to arise; the uterus must then be receptive to the fertilized egg which will grow in the womb nourished by the mother's blood and protected by the amniotic fluid. Pregnancy is considered a yin state as women generally become more receptive, introspective and emotional, completely consumed by the tiny life developing within. To the foetus, utterly dependant on its mother, gestation is yang.

Acupuncture (see page 24) is a tried and tested means of helping couples become pregnant. Rather than predicting fertility using the days of the woman's typical cycle, many Chinese physicians use Basal Body Temperature or BBT. BBT rises approximately 0.5 °C (1°F) at the onset of ovulation, remaining at this level until the day before menstruation begins. If the woman becomes pregnant, BBT remains elevated.

BABY GENDER PREDICTION CHART

MONTH OF CONCEPTION

AGE	JAN	FEB	MAR	APR	MAY	JUN	JUL	AUG	SEP	OCT	NOV	DEC
18	X	O	X	O	O	O	O	O	O	O	O	O
19	O	X	O	X	X	O	O	X	O	O	X	X
20	X	O	X	O	O	O	O	O	O	X	O	O
21	O	X	X	X	X	X	X	X	X	X	X	X
22	X	O	O	X	O	X	X	O	X	X	X	X
23	O	O	O	X	O	O	X	X	X	O	O	X
24	O	X	X	O	O	O	X	X	O	O	X	O
25	X	O	X	O	X	O	X	O	X	O	O	O
26	O	O	O	O	O	X	X	X	X	O	X	X
27	X	X	O	O	X	O	X	X	O	X	O	O
28	O	O	O	X	X	O	X	O	X	X	O	X
29	X	O	X	X	O	X	X	O	X	O	X	X
30	O	O	X	O	X	O	O	O	O	O	O	O
31	O	O	O	O	X	O	X	X	O	X	X	X
32	O	X	X	O	X	O	O	X	O	O	X	O
33	X	O	O	X	X	O	X	O	X	O	O	X
34	O	O	X	X	O	X	O	O	X	O	X	X
35	O	X	O	X	O	X	O	X	O	O	X	O
36	O	X	O	O	O	X	O	O	X	X	X	O
37	X	X	O	X	X	X	O	X	X	O	O	O
38	O	O	O	X	O	X	X	O	X	X	O	X
39	X	X	O	X	X	X	O	X	O	O	X	O
40	O	O	O	X	O	X	O	X	O	X	X	O
41	X	X	O	X	O	O	X	X	O	X	O	X
42	O	X	X	O	O	O	O	O	X	O	X	O
43	X	O	X	X	O	O	O	X	X	X	O	O
44	O	X	X	X	O	X	O	O	X	O	X	O
45	X	O	X	O	X	X	O	X	O	X	O	X

O-Boy   X-Girl

A further indication of fertility is the change in the fertile mucous secretions around the cervical opening of the vaginal canal. Mucous is dry and scarce immediately after menstruation, becoming wet and sticky prior to ovulation and turning thin and elastic at ovulation—exactly when the woman is most fertile.

For those couples which do become pregnant the Baby Gender Prediction Chart, resurrected from the royal tomb outside Beijing hundreds of years ago, is much used by TCM practitioners (see previous page). The original chart was kept in Beijing's Institute of Science and was later adapted to the Western calendar. It is said to accurately predict a baby's gender in 90% of cases. All that is required is the woman's age at conception and the month of conception.

The Menstrual Cycle

Governed by the earth element, a regular menstrual cycle—on time and relatively pain-free—is a sign that blood and *Qi* circulation are in order. Anything other than this is indicative of disharmony, either hormonally related or the result of external factors like stress, diet or emotional upset.

PHASE I: MENSTRUATION
Yin • BBT: low (36.2-$36.5°C$/97.1-$97.7°F$)

According to Western thinking, a decrease in the levels of oestrogen and progesterone results in the shedding of the endometrial (uterine) lining. Chinese medicine purports that blood flow through the smaller vessels of the endometrium (lining of the uterus) should be smooth and relatively pain-free. If flow is disrupted, the typical symptoms of dysmenorrhoea (painful menstruation) will be experienced. As menstrual blood is a direct reflection of each woman's health, blood that is of poor colour and consistency suggests possible

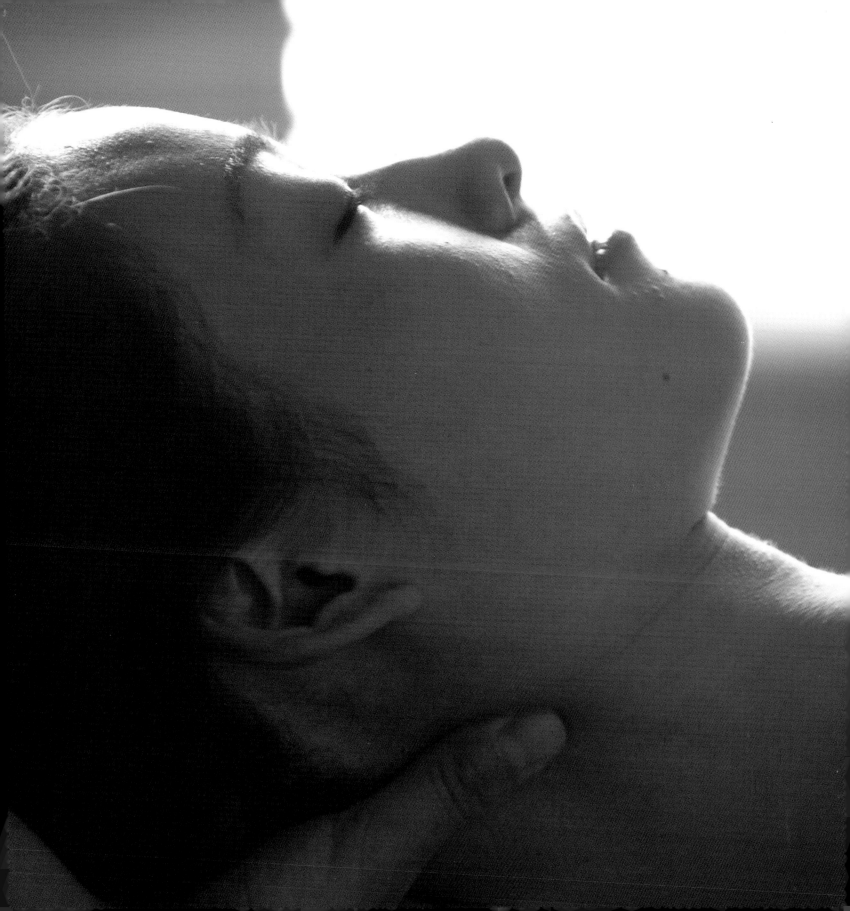

fertility issues. The Chinese use the herbs *chuan xiong (Radix ligustici wallichii)* and *dang gui (Radix angelica sinensis)* in this first phase.

Foods to eat: Fresh ginger, Chinese wine or red wine, sunflower seeds, celery, Chinese chives and coriander, chicken, mutton, pork, polished rice and foods rich in magnesium like green vegetables, cereals, almonds and Brazil nuts.

Foods to restrict: All refined sugars, animal fats, dairy products and trans-fatty acids in deep fried foods and some margarines.

Recommended Chinese herbal formulations:
Persica Carthamus Four Substance Decoction Teapills (Tao Hong Si Wu Tang) from Plum Flower Brand.
Dosage: Eight pills, three times a day during menstruation (may be increased to 12 pills, three times a day if necessary). Prohibited during pregnancy.

Jia Wei Xiao Yao Wan from Tong Ren Tang.
Dosage: Contents of one sachet (i.e. 100 pills), two to three times a day during menstruation.

Bak Foong Pills from Eu Yan Sang.
Dosage: To be determined by a Chinese medicine physician.

PHASE II: POST-MENSTRUATION
Yin • BBT: low (36.2-36.5°C/97.1-97.7°F)

In Western thinking, during the post-menstruation phase, the follicles develop and the ovaries secrete oestrogen under the influence of FSH (Follicle Stimulating Hormone). The Chinese believe that the objective during this phase is to strengthen blood and yin after the

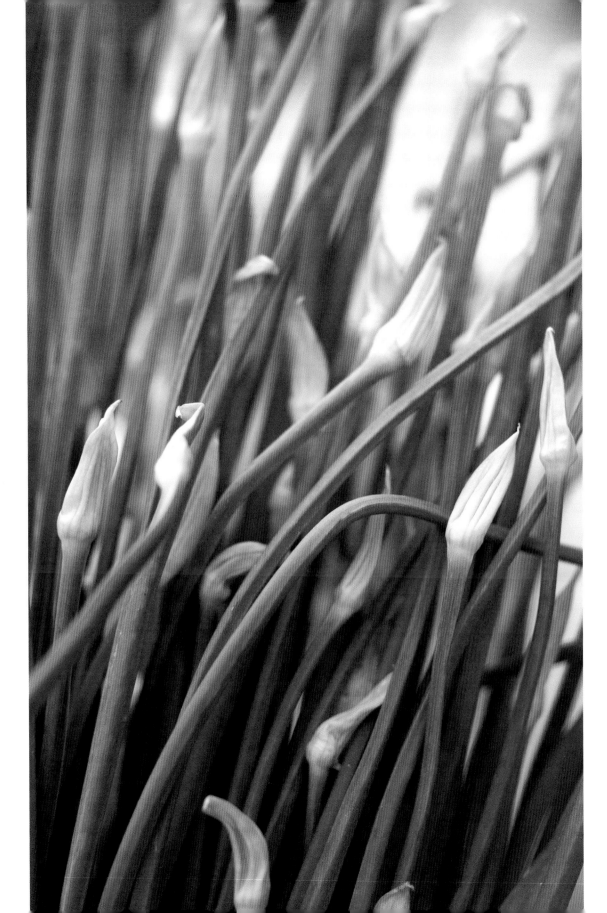

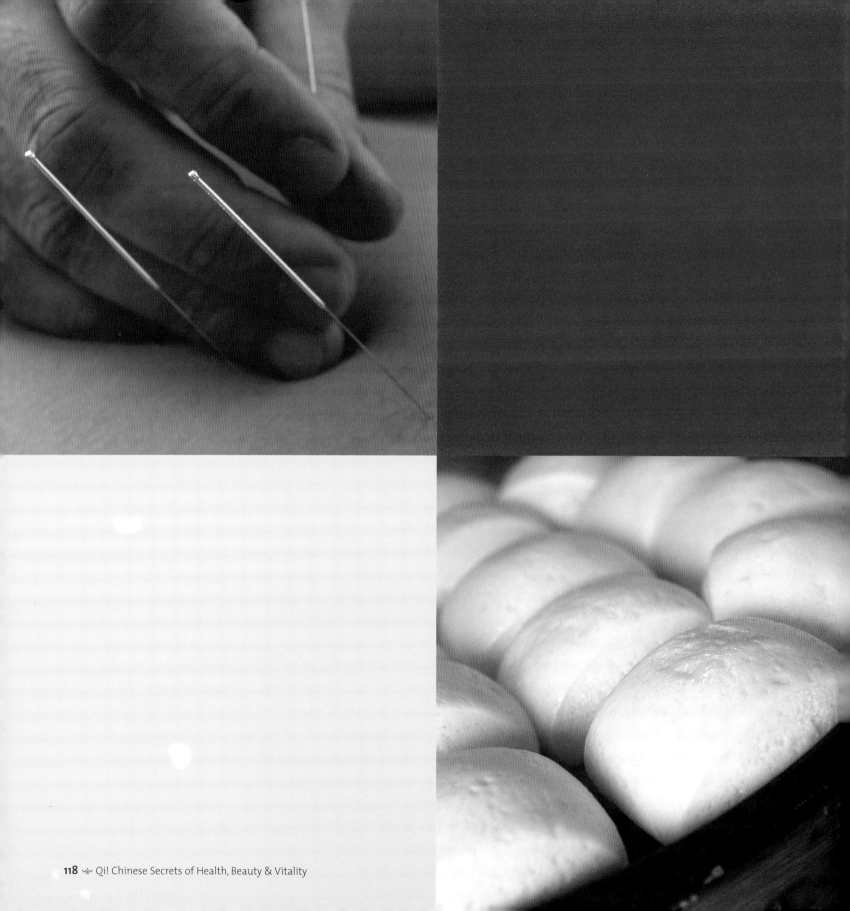

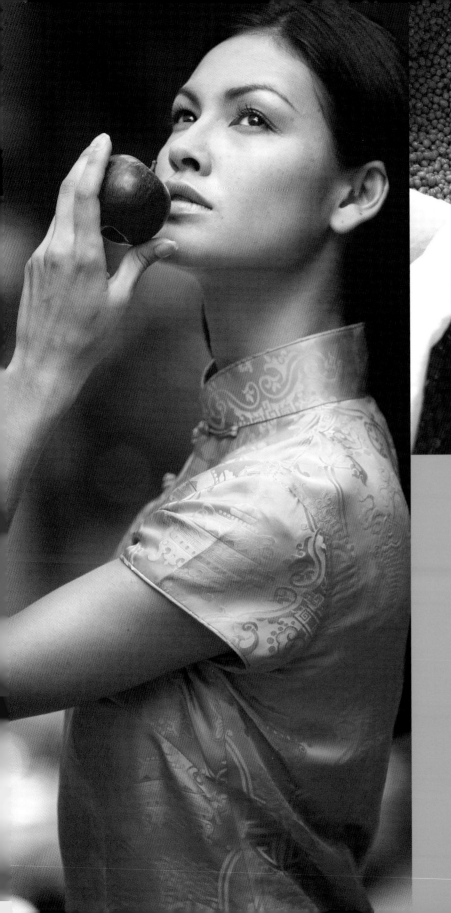
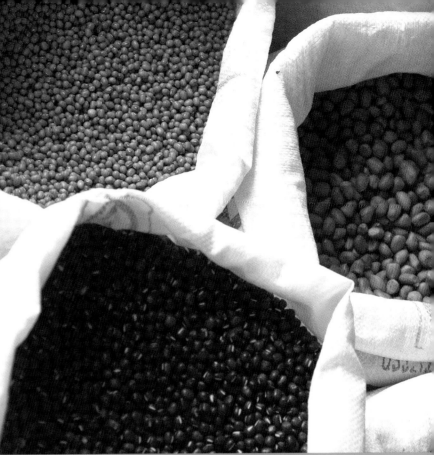

losses of menstruation thereby ensuring the fertile cervical mucus is thick and creamy in anticipation of pregnancy. Blockage or dysfunction in the uterus or in the flow of *Qi* can lead to breakthrough bleeding and conception difficulties. Herbs used during this time include *shu di huang (Radix rehmanniae glutinosae conquitae)* and *bai shao (Radix paeonia lactiflorae albae)*. Acupuncture is also thought to help regulate the circulation of *Qi* and blood, removing any obstruction.

Foods to eat: Fibre-rich foods like wholegrain breads, cereals, brown rice and whole-wheat pasta.

Recommended Chinese herbal formulations:

Six Flavour Teapills (Liu Wei Di Huang Wan) from Plum Flower Brand.

Dosage: Eight tablets, three times a day from the end of menstruation to the start of ovulation.

Motherhood Formula (Tiao Jing Cuyun Wan) from Tong Ren Tang.

Dosage: 25-50 pills twice a day, starting on the fifth day of the menstrual cycle, for 20 days. If there is no menstrual cycle, take for 20 days each month. Take consecutively for three months or as prescribed by a Chinese medicine physician.

Bak Foong Pills from Eu Yan Sang.

Dosage: To be determined by a Chinese medicine physician.

PHASE III: OVULATION
Yang • BBT: high (BBT rises by 0.3-0.5°C/0.5-0.9°F)

According to Western medicine, the ovum is released from the follicle during ovulation, leaving a "crater" which later becomes the corpus luteum. The Chinese believe that the transition between yin and yang at ovulation regulates the menstrual cycle. Characterized by an increase in body temperature (to warm the uterus in anticipation of pregnancy), this change has several effects on the reproductive organs. The cervical mucus becomes thin and elastic, providing the sperm with a clear thoroughfare. While in the endometrium, blood vessels grow and thicken. Herbs thought to aid this transition are *du zhong (Cortex eucommiae ulimoidis)* and *bai zhu (Rhizoma atractylodis macrocephalae)*.

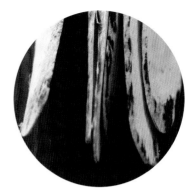

Foods to choose: Dark green vegetables, ginger, fresh ling, water chestnuts, mussels and Vitamin E-rich foods like wheatgerm, safflower oil and sprouting seeds.

Recommended Chinese herbal formulations:

You Gui Teapills from Plum Flower Brand.

Dosage: Eight pills, three times a day if needed during ovulation.

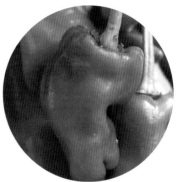

Motherhood Formula (Tiao Jing Cuyun Wan) from Tong Ren Tang.

Dosage: 25-50 pills twice a day.

Bak Foong Pills from Eu Yan Sang.

Dosage: To be determined by a Chinese medicine physician.

PHASE IV: PRE-MENSTRUATION
Yang • BBT: high (36.8°C/98.2°F)

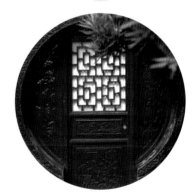

Western science notes that the corpus luteum continues to grow and secrete progesterone during this phase. The noticeable craving for sweet and processed foods typically experienced a few days prior to menstruation should stop once core body temperature drops by 0.3°C 24 hours before menstruation begins. Chinese medicine employs herbs such as *chai hu (Radix bupleuri)* and *bai shao (Radix paeonia lactiflorae albae)* during this phase. It also states that

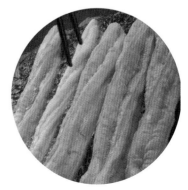

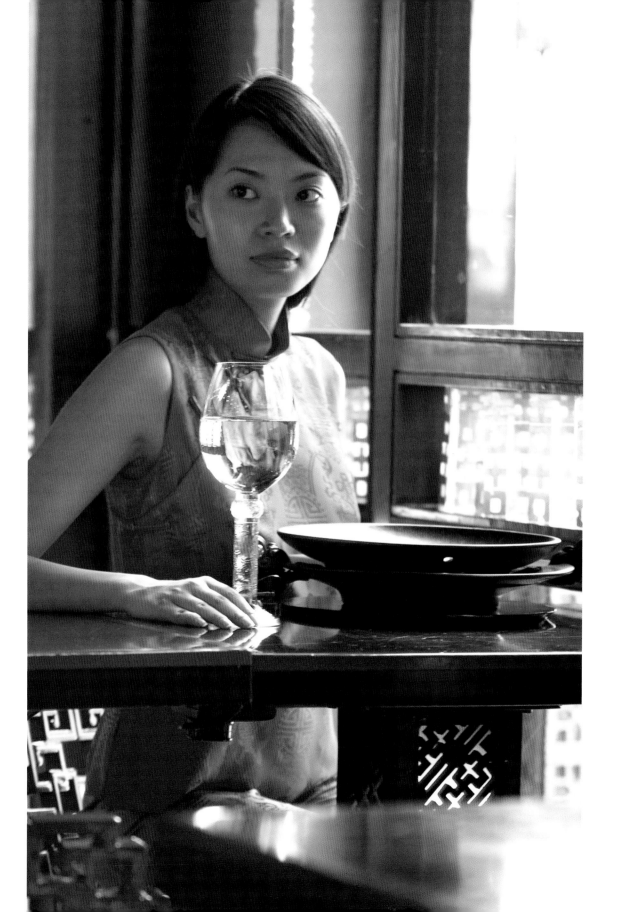

many of the unpleasant symptoms associated with pre-menstruation can be alleviated by simple dietary changes such as avoiding sweet foods and choosing more pungent flavours to disperse blood and *Qi*.

Foods to choose: Fibre-rich whole foods like brown rice and rye, leafy greens, celery, cucumber, eggs, walnuts, ginger, yellow soybeans, mung beans, corn and eggplants.

Foods to restrict: Wheat-based foods (being sour they tend to constrict blood flow), salty foods, processed and refined sugars and trans-fatty acids.

Recommended Chinese herbal formulations:
Added Ingredients Free and Relaxed Teapills (Jia Wei Xiao Yao Wan) from Plum Flower Brand.
Dosage: Eight tablets, three times a day when premenstrual symptoms occur (can be increased to 12 tablets, three times a day, if needed).

Australian Natural Deer Velvet Powder Capsules (Lu Rong Jiao Nang) from Tong Ren Tang.
Dosage: Four capsules a day.

Motherhood Formula (Tiao Jing Cuyun Wan) from Tong Ren Tang.
Dosage: 25-50 pills twice a day.

Bak Foong Pills from Eu Yan Sang.
Dosage: To be determined by a Chinese medicine physician.

Premenstrual Tension

About one week before menstruation begins, PMT can produce mood swings from depression to irritability and anger; tender breasts; exhaustion; a bloated stomach; skin eruptions; and changes in bowel habits and libido. For millions of women these symptoms subside as soon as menstruation begins.

In Chinese medicine the root cause of many of these seemingly unrelated conditions is liver *Qi* stagnation which can be caused by a range of factors including stress, environmental toxins, drugs and the natural rhythms of a woman's BBT. If unresolved, liver *Qi* stagnation gives rise to blood stagnation, tension in the muscles and along the liver meridian (breasts) and the other symptoms described above.

The goal of Chinese therapy is simply to move *Qi* and blood. This is done through eating the recommended foods listed below. Chinese herbal medicines and tonics are very helpful but can take up to four months for maximum effect. Acupuncture starting midway through ovulation is commonly used as a preventive measure to realign hormones, paving the way to a smoother, more pain-free cycle. Aerobic exercises involving abdominal breathing, like *tai chi*, yoga or swimming, further relieve discomfort. Regular sex is also a noted oestrogen balancer.

EATING FOR A SMOOTHER CYCLE

Eat regularly to keep blood-sugar levels more evenly balanced. To alleviate mood swings cut sugar and other refined foods and stimulants like coffee, tea and alcohol. Think unrefined cereals, vegetables, nuts and fruits.

As many women experience a premenstrual tightening of the diaphragm area, pineapple which is rich in the enzyme bromelain helps ease contractions. Green tea or a cup of warm water with a teaspoon of aloe vera juice helps soothe and calm both body and mind. Fennel nurtures the blood and is ideally taken as a drink (half to one litre a day) mixed with carrot juice. Supplements of Vitamin-B Complex and magnesium (both needed for the production of the "feel-good hormones" dopamine and noradrenaline in the brain) help you feel brighter, more focused and better able to deal with stress.

Soya (as in tofu, miso and beancurd) is packed with phytoesterols, a well-recognized oestrogen balancer. Oestrogen is thought to act as a mild antidepressant, and when levels are low (as they generally are towards the end of the cycle) women can feel completely drained. Also during this time, progesterone levels are raised which makes tiredness worse.

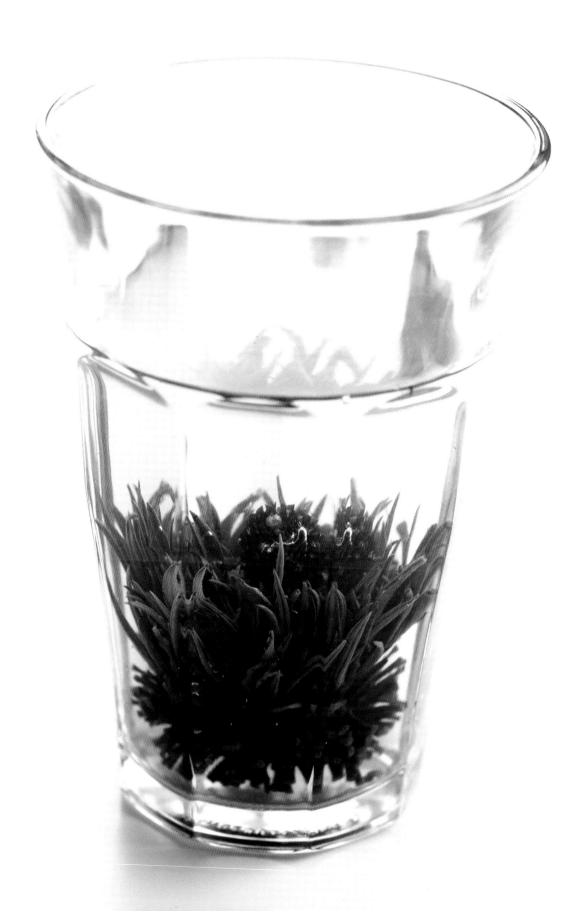

- ✤ **Eat more wholegrains, green vegetables, wholewheat cereals and fruit.**

- ✤ **Avoid sugar, refined carbohydrates, caffeine and alcohol.**

- ✤ **Eat more soya in its various guises (tofu, beancurd, miso).**

- ✤ **Drink green tea.**

- ✤ **Take 1-2 tbsp flaxseeds or linseeds.**

Recommended supplements:

The following supplements should be taken for 10-14 days before menstruation begins.

- ✤ **Vitamin B6:** 100-200mg or B-complex vitamins with a minimum of 50mg vitamin B6.

- ✤ **Magnesium:** 200-800mg elemental magnesium.

- ✤ **Evening Primrose Oil (EPO) or Starflower Oil:** Both rich in omega-6 fatty acids with a recommended dose being 1g of EPO or 500mg Starflower Oil three times a day.

Aromatherapy oils:

- ✤ **Geranium, marjoram, lavender and clary sage.**

- ✤ **Tarragon** (12 drops in ¹/₂ cup oil) massaged on the lower abdomen warms and disperses *Qi*.

FLUID RETENTION

For most women it is the interruption in the flow of *Qi* commonly seen premenstrually that leads to an accumulation of fluid and the symptoms of bloating and fluid retention. Other possible causes include hormonal imbalance, diet (food intolerance or an excess of raw and cold foods which slows digestion putting unnecessary strain on the organs) or a build-up of "bad" bacteria like *Candida albicans* in the bowel (which can be exacerbated by hormonal fluctuations). Chinese practitioners generally prescribe herbs such as ginseng or *ren shen (Radix panax ginseng)* and *bai shao (Radix paeoniae lactiflorae albae)* to realign hormones naturally, thereby reducing the symptoms of bloating. If bloating persists it is wise to seek professional advice but some useful measures in keeping with Chinese medicine include:

- **Eat more warm and cooked foods.**
- **Reduce intake of dairy products.**
- **Potassium-rich foods like bananas, tomatoes, watermelon, potatoes, green leafy vegetables, celery, artichoke, asparagus, parsley and watercress help reduce sodium levels, thereby eliminating excess water from the body.**
- **Drink chamomile tea (it is a mild diuretic).**
- **If bloating is bacteria-related, a daily dose of probiotic or "good" bacteria (acidophilus or bifidus) taken via live yoghurt, a probiotic supplement or unleavened wheatcakes helps repopulate the gut with healthy cultures.**
- **If bloating is food-related, the most common offenders are wheat, corn and dairy products. Remove these foods individually from your diet. If you feel better, you have found the culprit.**
- **Drink at least one litre of water each day.**
- **Avoid carbonated drinks.**
- **Relax more, especially when eating. The connection between the mind and gut is huge.**
- **Lymphatic drainage massage therapy helps clear the build-up of toxins and fluid from the body.**

Recommended Chinese herbal formulations:

Free and Easy Wanderer Teapills (Xiao Yao Wan) from Plum Flower Brand.

Dosage: Eight tablets, three times a day when bloating symptoms first appear.

Liver Tonic and Digestive Aid (Jia Wei Xiao Yao Wan) from Tong Ren Tang.

Dosage: Contents of one 6g sachet (100 pills), two to three times a day, when symptoms occur.

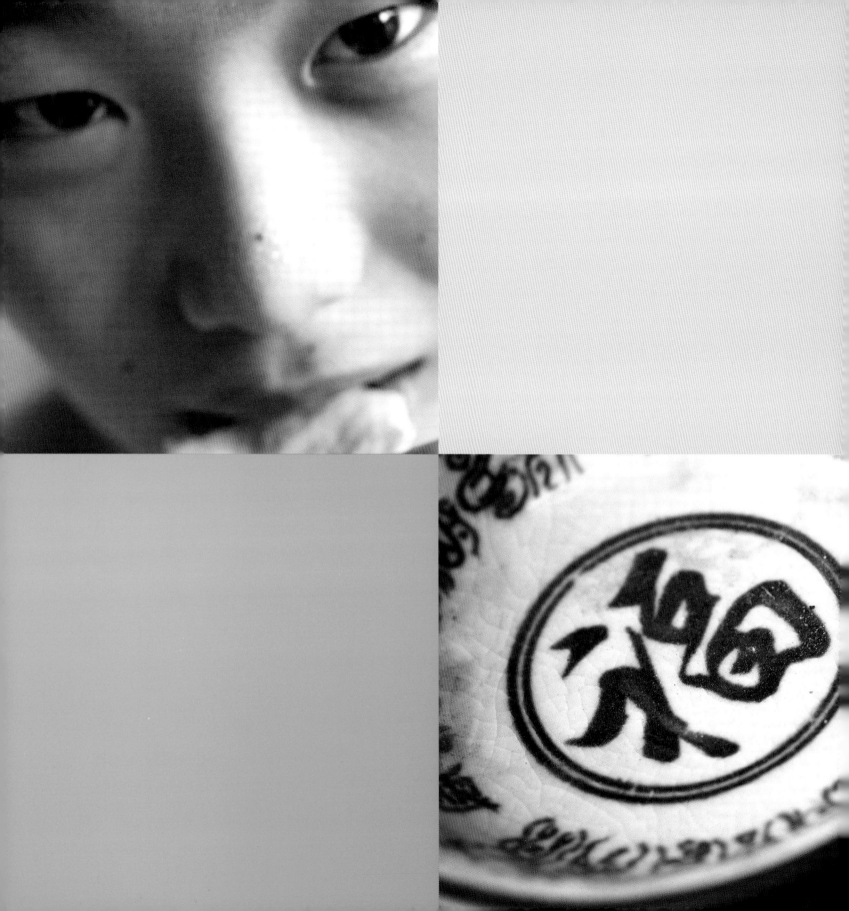

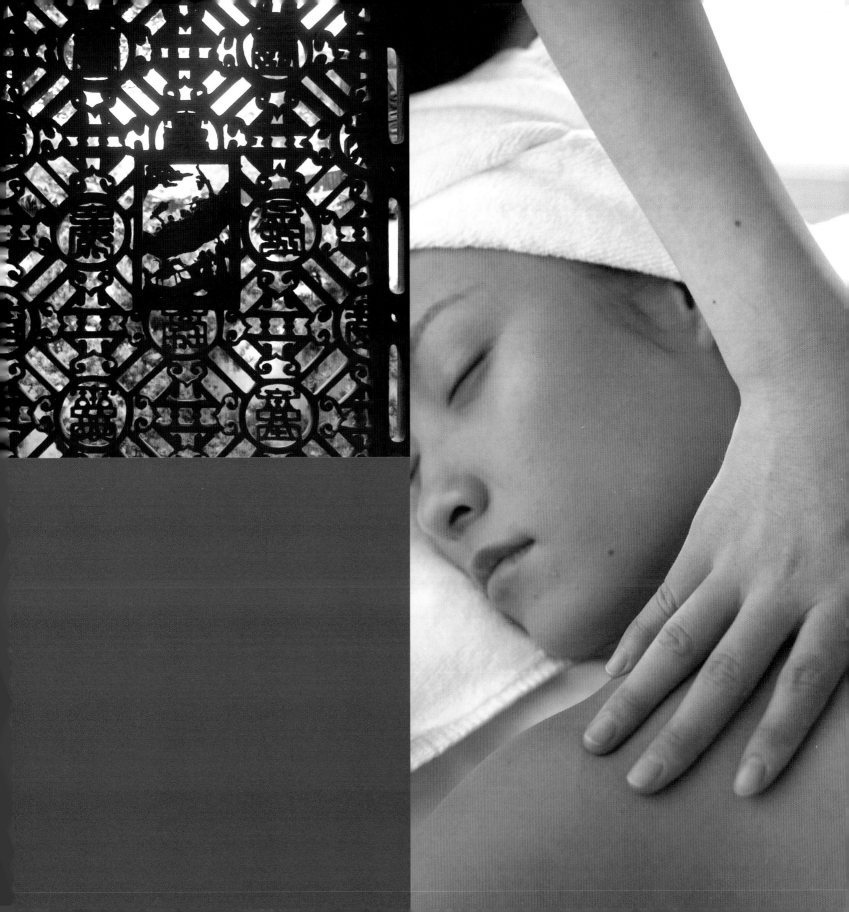

Boosting Fertility

"Life is warmth—if the womb or uterus is too cold, life cannot arise."

—Fu Qing Zhi (18th century AD)

Chinese medicine has helped thousands of women worldwide conceive and deliver hearty, healthy babies. Planning a pregnancy is the ideal time to invest in your body—for both you and your baby. Stress, overwork and smoking are major factors affecting fertility in both men and women, depleting the vital essence and causing tiredness, decreased libido and infertility.

Ideally, any changes in diet and lifestyle should be made at least three months before the intended time of conception. As an optimum level of body fat (20-26%) helps maintain regular hormonal activity, both overweight and underweight women can have a more difficult time conceiving and carrying a healthy baby to term.

As seen with The Menstrual Cycle (page 114), a woman's most fertile time is characterized by the transition from yin to yang and the concurrent rise in body temperature and change in mucous consistency which generally happens between days 10 and 16 of the average cycle. To maximize the chances of pregnancy, body temperature must remain raised for as long as possible. Acupuncture the day before ovulation (to physically move blood to the uterus) and four days later (to promote implantation) is thought to greatly increase the chances of conception.

To ensure an adequate supply of healthy sperm, Chinese experts recommend abstinence from sex for at least four days after monthly bleeding stops followed by sex every second day for eight consecutive days.

FOOD AND FERTILITY

Warm and cooked foods promote a smoother flow of *Qi* and blood to the uterus to warm the reproductive organs. Meals should be packed with cooked fresh vegetables, fruits, wholegrains and lean proteins, while coffee, alcohol, sugar, wheat, processed and fried foods should be avoided or at least reduced substantially.

If the uterus is "cold" and/or "damp", Chinese herbs such as *tu si zi (Semen custcutae)* and *xu duan (Radix dipsaci)* are usually prescribed. Foods like green raspberries, cinnamon, kidney

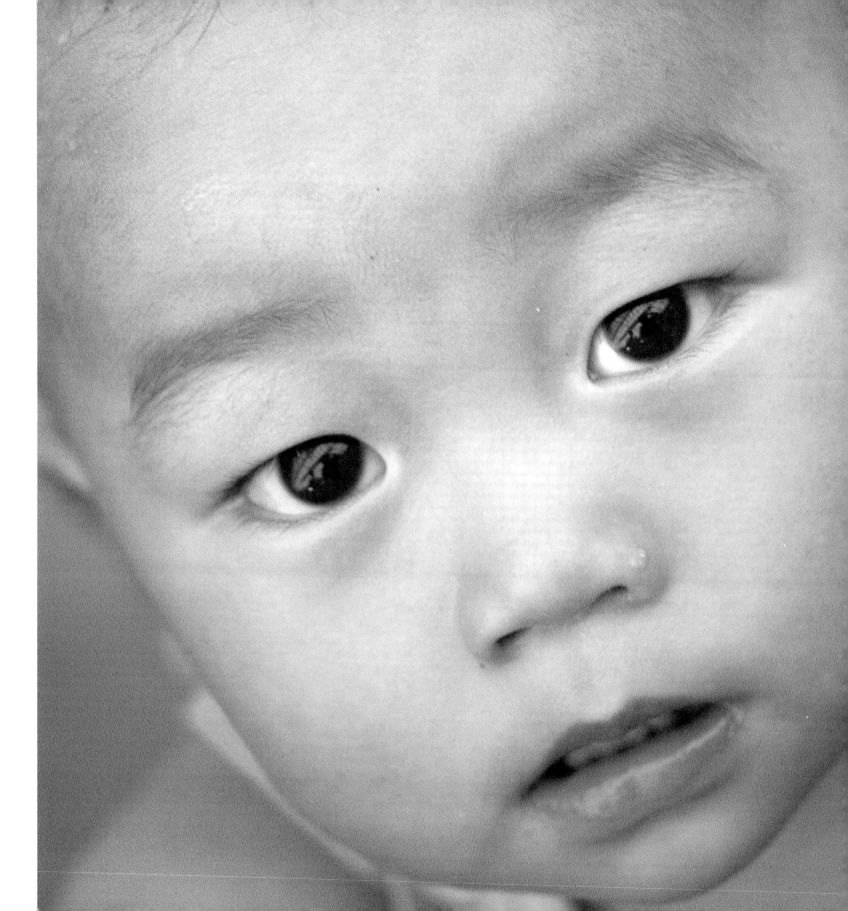

beans, sheep's milk, sardines, shrimp, and red and black dates are thought to warm the area, making it more conducive to accepting a fertilized egg. The following food elements are particularly important.

Zinc: Zinc nourishes the liver and enriches the kidneys. It is also essential for healthy sperm development so men should eat more zinc-rich foods like venison, shellfish (especially oysters) and red meat (especially organ meats). Both caffeine and cigarettes significantly reduce the uptake of zinc in the body and are ideally avoided.

Folic acid: A blood nourisher for the mother, folic acid is also essential for the healthy development of the neural tube which forms the baby's spinal cord and develops during the first three months of pregnancy. Experts recommend a supplement of 400 micrograms of folic acid daily before and during the first trimester of pregnancy. Folic acid-rich foods like spinach and other leafy greens, beetroot, yeast extract, wholemeal bread and fortified breakfast cereals are ideal for mothers-to-be.

Iron: Iron is essential for healthy blood and muscles. Iron-deficiency anaemia is especially common in women (most notably those with heavy periods) and can adversely affect their ability to conceive. As with all nutrients, iron relies on a healthy gut for absorption and women with digestive problems or chronic constipation tend to be at a greater risk of deficiency. If iron deficiency is suspected a course of supplements (50-100mg iron taken daily with food) along with a supplement of Vitamin C is recommended.

Recommended Chinese herbal formulations:
You Gui Teapills from Plum Flower Brand.
Dosage: Eight tablets, three times a day, for about 15 days starting mid-cycle (can be increased to 12 tablets, three times a day if necessary).

Motherhood Formula (Tiao Jing Cuyun Wan) from Tong Ren Tang.
Dosage: 25-50 pills twice a day, starting on the fifth day of the menstural cycle, for 20 days.

Bak Foong Pills from Eu Yan Sang.
Dosage: To be determined by a Chinese medicine physician.

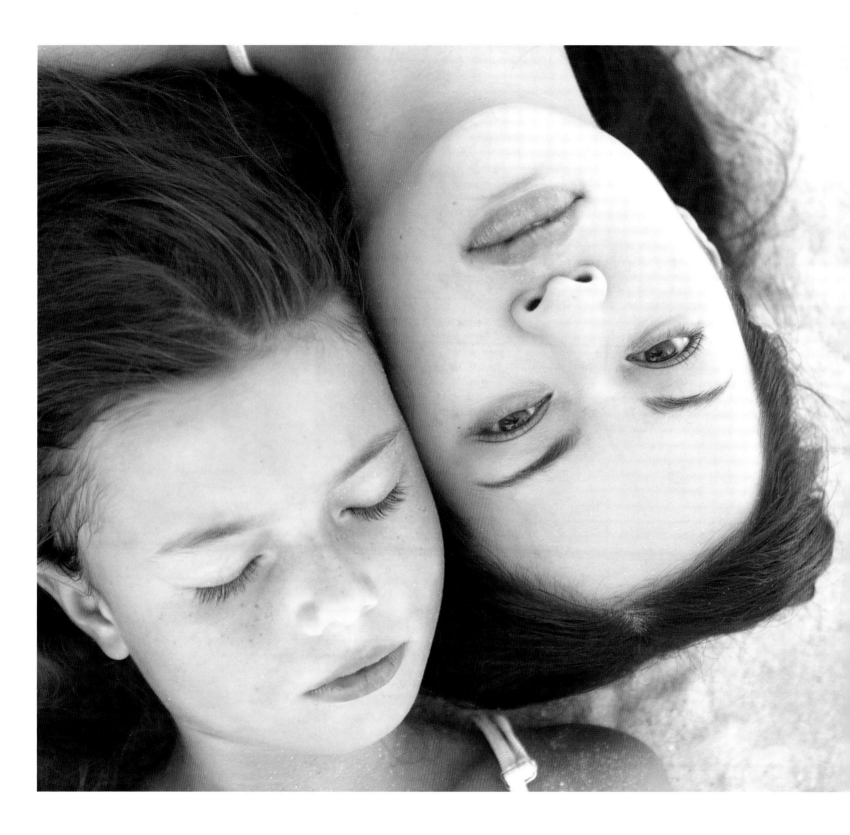

Menopause

Menopause is defined as the permanent cessation of menstruation which in TCM begins around the seventh of the seven-year cycles (i.e. about 49 years) of a woman's life. Perimenopause, the two to eight years of fluctuating hormones which result in irregular menstruation leading up to menopause, is considered by TCM as the first stage in this natural progression. The kidneys are seen to gradually become exhausted with age until the menstrual essence (*tian gui*) is depleted and menopause occurs.

With the average life expectancy of women in developed countries being 85, most women will experience some or all of the conditions related to menopause for up to one-third of their lives. These conditions include hot flushes, psychosomatic illnesses, genital

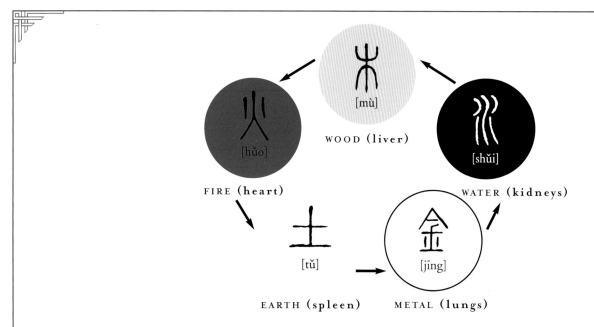

[mù]

WOOD (liver)

[huǒ]

FIRE (heart)

[shuǐ]

WATER (kidneys)

[tǔ]

EARTH (spleen)

[jing]

METAL (lungs)

THE FIVE ELEMENTS' NURTURING CYCLE

As well as controlling one another (see page 18), the elements (and their associated organs) support one another, as shown above. Thus if one organ (e.g. lungs) is unwell, a tonic may be recommended for its nurturing organ (e.g. spleen). This nurturing cycle is also reflected in the seasons, with the water phase of winter a yin time of reflection, waiting for spring. The wood phase of spring signifies the birth of new life, before moving to the hot yang of summer. Fire represents yang's peak before moving to the earth phase of maturation through autumn's metal, with yin on the incline as winter approaches. Symbols courtesy of Banyan Tree Spa Shanghai.

changes and osteoporosis.

Hot flushes, which may be accompanied by insomnia, restlessness, irritability and emotional stress, occur in 80% of postmenopausal women. The visible flushing of blood in the face, neck and upper chest is followed by an increase in temperature and profuse sweating, typically lasting for four minutes.

Genital changes affect about 20% of postmenopausal women. Reduced oestrogen may result in vaginal dryness, which in turn causes painful intercourse, reduced libido, and an increased risk of infection in the genito-urinary region.

Osteoporosis is a condition of brittle and fragile bones (*guwei*), which in menopause is caused by hormonal changes. Bone fractures are one of the main problems of osteoporosis.

The water element associated with the kidneys inhibits or controls excess fire in the heart (see the Five Elements' Controlling Cycle, page 18). When the interaction between the kidneys and the heart is adversely affected, hot flushes, heart palpitations, psychological and emotional distress and other menopausal symptoms may occur. Kidney water also moistens or nurtures the wood element of the liver, as shown in the Five Elements' Nurturing Cycle (opposite). When this supportive relationship between the kidneys and the liver breaks down, liver function is impaired. Thus, TCM seeks to enrich the kidneys which in turn benefits both the heart and liver.

Acupuncture (taken over a few months) has been found to relieve hot flushes, headaches and osteoporosis as well as emotional stress and tension.

Many menopuasal changes are a result of a decrease in the production of the hormone oestrogen. Chemicals called phytoestrogens, occurring in some plants, may act like oestrogen in the body. Thus, a diet high in phytoestrogen sources such as soybeans, soy flour, tofu, Mexican yams, red clover and linseed oil is recommended during menopause. Other dietary measures are in the sidebar (right).

Recommended supplements:
· **Vitamin E**: 100-500mg a day (seek medical advice if you have high blood pressure).
· **Vitamin C with Bioflavonoids**: see manufacturer's recommended dosages.
· **Evening Primrose Oil (EPO)**: 1g three times a day.

Foods that nourish the kidneys include:
Fruit, nuts and vegetables: adzuki beans, apples, apricots, bananas, broccoli, cabbage, Chinese cabbage, cashews, celery, coconut, corn, cucumber, eggplant, figs, grapefruit, green beans, kidney beans, lentils, lettuce, mandarins, papayas, parsnips, peanuts, potatoes, prunes, plums, snow peas, spinach, sweet potatoes, tomatoes, turnips, walnuts, watercress, watermelon, zucchini and other squashes.

Proteins: eggs, fish, lamb, pork, tofu and yoghurt.

Grains and seeds: barley, black sesame seeds, brown rice, flaxseeds, oats, sunflower seeds, walnuts and wild rice.

Other foods: basil, flaxeed oil, ginseng, honey, sesame oil and soy sauce.

See also pages 44-45 for other water element (Winter) foods.

Foods to reduce or avoid during menopause include: alcohol, coffee and other forms of caffeine, cured meats, dairy products (except yoghurt), fried, fatty, spicy and processed foods, and red meats other than those specified in Proteins (above).

Recommended Chinese herbal formulations:

Eight Flavour Rehmannia Teapills (Zhi Bai Di Huang Wan) from Plum Flower Brand. For hot flushes, lower back pain, night sweats, irritability, anxiety, insomnia, fluid retention and heart palpitations.
Dosage: Eight pills, three times a day.

Free and Easy Wanderer Plus Teapills (Jia Wei Xiao Yao San) combined with Calm Spirit Teapills (Gan Mai Da Zao Tang) from Plum Flower Brand. For depression.
Dosage: Eight pills of each, three times a day.

Free and Easy Wanderer Plus Teapills (Jia Wei Xiao Yao San) combined with Two Immortals Teapills (Er Xian Wan) from Plum Flower Brand. For high blood pressure, hot flushes, sweating, anxiety, irritability, fatigue, insomnia and heart palpitations.
Dosage: Eight pills of each, three times a day.

Abundant Yin Teapills (Da Bu Yin Wan) from Plum Flower Brand. For osteoporosis.
Dosage: Eight pills, three times a day.

Women's Treasure Pills (Kunbao Wan) from Tong Ren Tang. For hot flushes.
Dosage: 50 pills, twice a day.

Menoease Pills from Eu Yan Sang. For a variety of menopausal conditions.
Dosage: To be determined by a Chinese medicine practitioner.

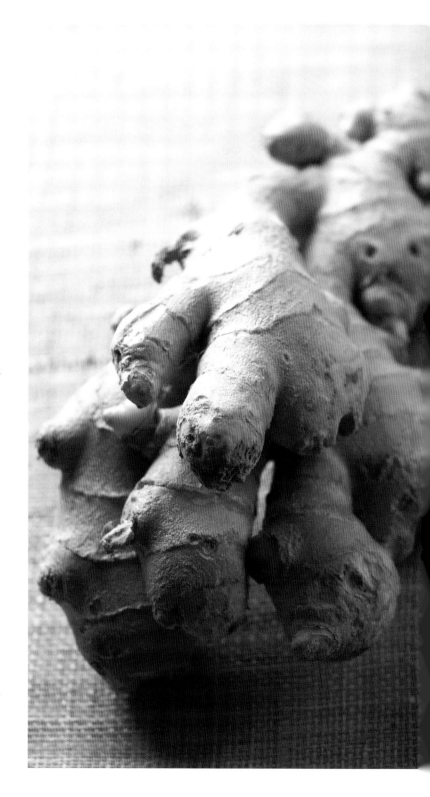

Recipes for Women's Health

Warming Soup

(1 serving)

Ideal for dysmennorrhoea. *Dang gui* is a blood tonic and mover. Mutton, ginger and chives are warm and assist in invigorating blood and dispelling "cold".

15g/0.6oz *dang gui*
250g/10oz mutton
60g/2.4oz fresh ginger
1 tbsp rice wine
1 tbsp Chinese chives
2 tsp peanut oil

Cut mutton into small pieces and fry in peanut oil. Add water, *dang gui*, fresh ginger and Chinese chives and simmer until cooked. Remove *dang gui*. Eat the mutton and drink the soup on the first day of menstruation.

Uterine Dysfunction Broth

(7 servings)

Promotes healthy circulation.

375g/15oz cuttlefish
75g/3oz *tao ren* (*Semen persicae*)
2 slices ginger
1 spring onion, shredded

Remove the "pen" from the cuttlefish, wash and cut into strips. Heat oil in wok; add cuttlefish, *tao ren*, ginger and water. Bring to the boil and reduce and simmer until cuttlefish is soft. Season with salt and sprinkle with shredded spring onion. Drink for one week from the end of menstruation.

Diuretic Tonic Soup

(4-6 servings)

Reduces bloating.

30g/1.2oz cornsilk
15g/0.6oz dry mandarin peel
1 slice fresh ginger
1 bunch fresh parsley
1 cup chopped celery
1/2 cup pearl barley
1 cup fresh chopped asparagus
30g/1.2oz *fu ling* (*Sclerotium poria cocos*)
8 cups vegetable stock

Place cornsilk, mandarin peel, ginger, parsley and fungus in a muslin bag. Add the asparagus and celery to barley and vegetable stock. Simmer for about 30 minutes. Serve warm.

Anaemia Tonic

(1 serving)

Ideal for anaemia, correcting menstrual disorders and improving the complexion. Red dates are better than black as only top quality fresh dates can be cured in the sun.

10 red dates
3g/0.1oz *dang gui*
1 cup water

Combine ingredients with a cup of water and heat over a low heat until reduced by half. Drink once daily for 10 days.

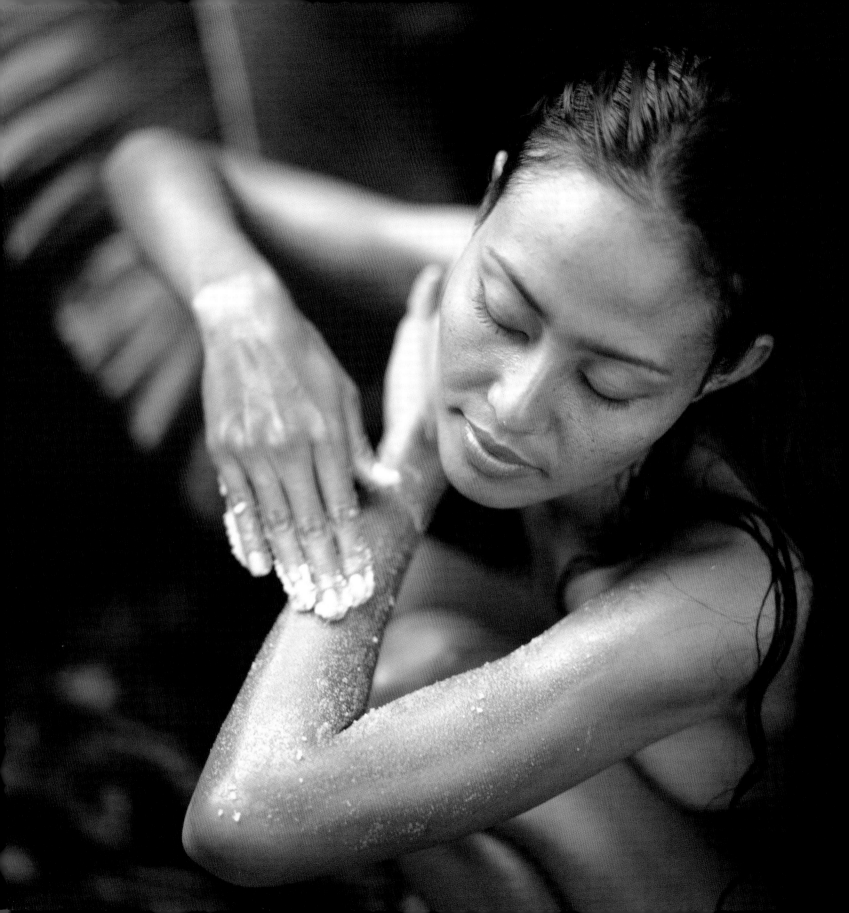

CHAPTER 5

Beauty, Chinese-style:
skin, hair and nails

"Female beauty was a subject of considerable interest to the Chinese from the earliest times … the catalogue of female attractions begins at the head and works downwards."

—Wolfram Eberhard, *A Dictionary of Chinese Symbols* (1986)

Qi for Beautiful Skin
Ruled by the lungs, skin achieves radiance through continuously

circulating *Qi*. This is promoted by a combination of eating with the seasons, exercise, adequate sleep and minimal stress. However, with constant damage from the sun, pollution and daily life, skin can be prone to dryness, sagging and wrinkles. Stress alone ages the skin dramatically as it becomes starved of *Qi* and nutrients and looks dull, tired and lifeless.

FACIAL REFLEX ZONES

"Before an omen arises, it's easy to take preventive measures."

– Lao Tzu, *Tao Te Ching* (c.1066-770BC)

In Chinese medicine the meridians are represented in zones of the face. To a trained Chinese medicine practitioner, imbalances in the body organs are revealed in the face. For example, female hormonal imbalance is indicated by irritation on the chin (the reflex zone for the kidneys which are partly responsible for oestrogen production). Corresponding facial zones and organs include:

Forehead: Intestine

Right cheek to base of face: Liver

Left cheek area: Lung

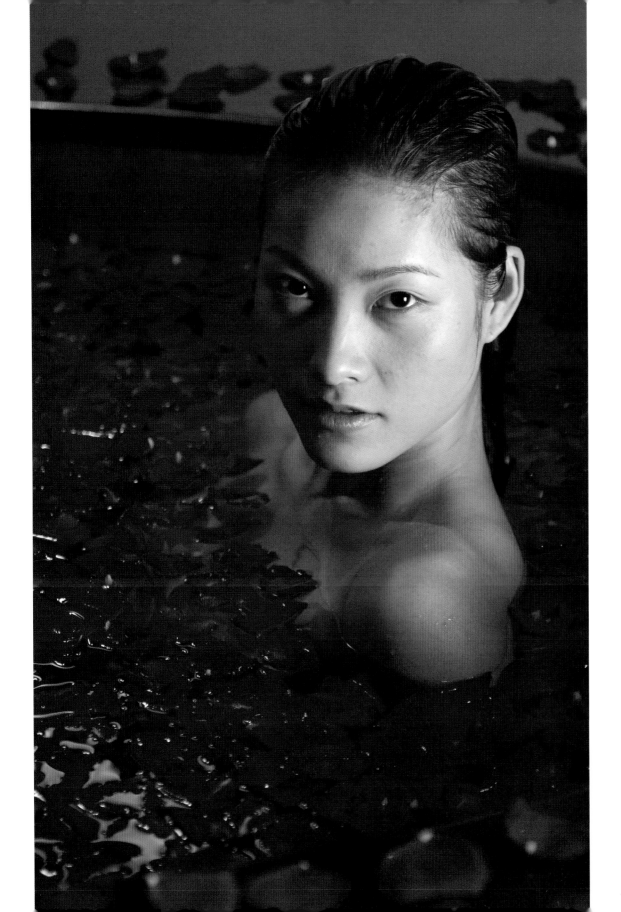

Nose: Heart

Mouth/Lips: Spleen

Chin: Kidneys

ENVIRONMENTAL HAZARDS

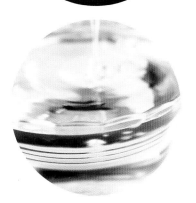

Nothing ages skin more than too much sun. While collagen provides the skin with a strong, firm texture and elastin maintains its resilience, ultraviolet radiation from the sun produces free radicals that destroy this network, accelerating premature ageing. Daily skin protection prevents damage and improves overall skin texture, reducing the appearance of wrinkles and lines.

Dietary culprits include alcohol and caffeine which disturb the body's natural balance, resulting in tired and dull-looking skin. Nicotene from cigarettes disrupts the flow of oxygen and *Qi* to the skin, leaving it dehydrated and lined.

PROTECT YOUR SKIN

* **Always use a sunscreen with a SPF (Sun Protection Factor) of 15 or higher and reapply frequently when in the sun.**
* **Use a moisturizer (specific to your skin type) morning and night.**
* **Wear a hat with a brim to protect the hair, scalp and face when directly exposed to the sun.**
* **Use nourishing and hydrating masks at least once a week.**

FEED YOUR SKIN

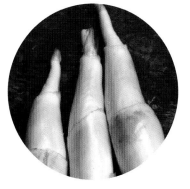

The Chinese have long realized that for healthy skin daily water and nourishment is an essential accompaniment to a good skincare routine. Eating and drinking well keeps the organs balanced and *Qi* flowing smoothly.

Water: One of the commonest causes of dehydrated skin is lack of fluid. Water is essential—taken either as cooling or warming drinks depending on whether you are a yang or a yin type.

Cold-water Oily Fish: Salmon, trout and tuna are packed with omega-3 fatty acids which strengthen the blood and give skin a fresh, soft look.

Fruit and Vegetables: The most nourishing varieties for the skin and lungs are apples, figs, berry fruits (especially raspberries and strawberries), apricots, Asian pears, Chinese red and black dates, papayas, adzuki beans, avocados, bean sprouts, broccoli and other dark green vegetables, carrots, celery, chickpeas, chicory, cucumbers, dandelion flowers, garlic, ginger, green beans, leeks, lentils, black beans, mung beans, onions, pumpkins, radishes, seaweed (especially arame, hijiki and kelp), spinach, sweet potatoes, water chestnuts, water-cress and squash.

Grains, Nuts and Seeds: Concentrate on black sesame seeds, brown rice, millet, sunflower seeds, whole grains, oats, walnuts and Brazil nuts.

Live Yoghurt: Yoghurt with active bacterial cultures helps maintain the body's natural acid mantle and combats the free radicals responsible for skin ageing.

Tofu and other soy-based foods contain phytoestrogens that are similar in structure to the female hormone oestrogen and help maintain moist, plump and firm skin.

Other Foods/Herbs: Cinnamon bark, bird's nest, goldenseal, honey, honeysuckle, licorice root, mint, nettles, peppermint, red clover, safflower oil, wood ear fungus, flaxseed oil, wheatgerm oil and bamboo shoots (pictured opposite).

Recommended Chinese herbal formulations:

Australian Natural Deer Velvet Powder Capsules (Lu Rong Jiao Nang) from Tong Ren Tang.
Dosage: Four capsules a day.

Eczema Herbal Treatment (Pi Fu Bing Xue Du Wan) from Tong Ren Tang.
Dosage: 10 to 20 pills, twice a day (or as recommended by a Chinese medicine practitioner).

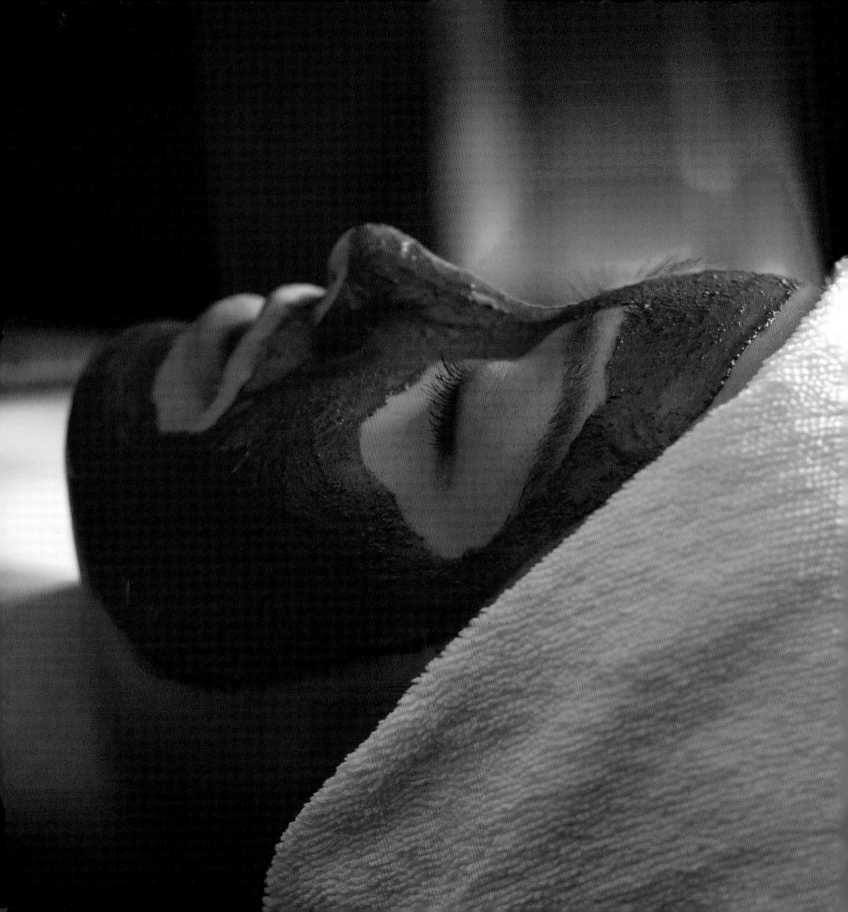

Yun Ji Pi Fu Paste from Tong Ren Tang.

Treatment: Cover skin with a thin layer from this 9g bottle, twice daily.

Bird's Nest products from Eu Yan Sang.

Dosage: At least twice a month.

OTHER SKINCARE ESSENTIALS

Exercise: Maintains a healthy flow of blood and *Qi* to the skin.

Sleep: Cellular repair of the skin is most active while we sleep.

Rest and Relaxation: Regular massage, rest and relaxation helps maintain internal balance and stress-free skin.

Massage: Acupressure and other facial massage therapies improve the flow of blood and *Qi* to the face, leaving it hydrated and glowing.

Essential Oils: To maintain a healthy glow use the essential oils outlined for your skin type (see below). When massaged onto the skin, they reach the inner cells, stimulating circulation and increasing the flow of *Qi*.

OILY SKIN

Oily skin is most commonly seen in Asians. Although fortunate to avoid fine lines and wrinkles, those with an oily complexion are more prone to acne, enlarged pores and blemishes. The goal of Chinese medicine is to regulate oil production and calm the skin and internal organs.

Essential Oils for Oily Skin: Lavender, lemon, basil, juniper, geranium and ylang ylang.

Do:

⊕ **Cleanse face twice a day with an alcohol-free liquid cleanser.**

⊕ **Choose oil-free or oil-in-water moisturizer.**

Create Your Own Face Oil
Add 25 drops of essential oil (specific to your skin type) to 25g/1 oz of almond or vegetable-base oil (sesame oil for dry skin). Dab a few drops in your hand, add a sprinkle of water and apply to moist skin. If using on the body, add 10 drops of essential oil to the base oil and apply directly to moistened skin.

- Use oil-free or oil-blotting foundation.
- Use oil-free sunscreen (SPF15 or higher) daily and reapply frequently especially when in the sun.

Don't:
- Overscrub the skin—oil is a protective barrier.
- Cleanse more than twice a day.
- Use powder to soak oil as it gives the skin a chalky appearance.

ACNE

A direct result of excess oil secretion on the skin's surface, acne is more commonly seen in hot yang types especially during the adolescent years. It can also arise or be exacerbated by hormonal or dietary imbalance, emotional upset, radical climate changes and poor hygiene.

Eating bamboo shoots (available in cans, sliced or in chunks) helps detoxify the skin but can cause bumps to erupt. Herbs that help relieve acne include honeysuckle, ginseng and dandelion flowers which are brewed and drunk as teas. A face mask of aloe vera gel and ginseng applied topically helps clear heat-induced blemishes. If you are prone to acne breakouts, it is best to avoid fried and spicy foods.

DRY SKIN

Women experiencing menopause and those prone to hormonal irregularities or menstrual problems often have dry skin, hair and eyes and an overall dehydrated countenance. For these women the nourishing qualities of yang foods, herbs and drinks will invigorate and revitalize the body.

Skin that is dry produces less oil and is therefore more prone to fine lines. Adzuki beans, papaya, ginseng, *dang gui*, honey, black sesame seeds, sunflower seeds, soy-based foods, flaxseeds, Chinese wolfberries, ginger and jelly textured foods (e.g. Royal Jelly, bird's nest, gelatin) all help plump the skin leaving it moisturized, hydrated and radiant.

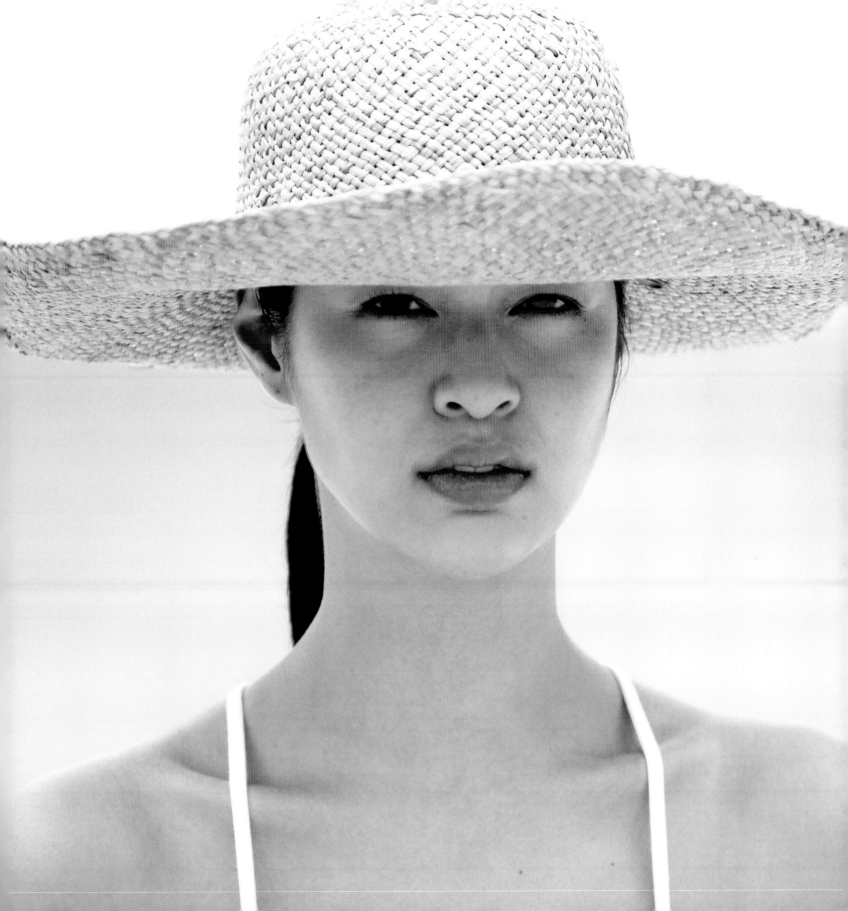

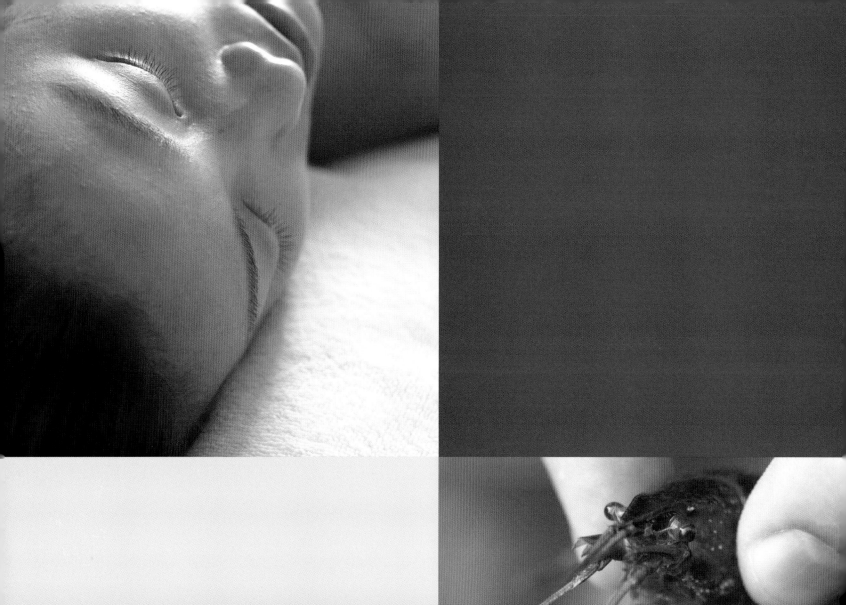
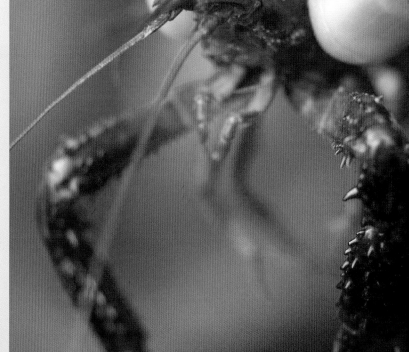

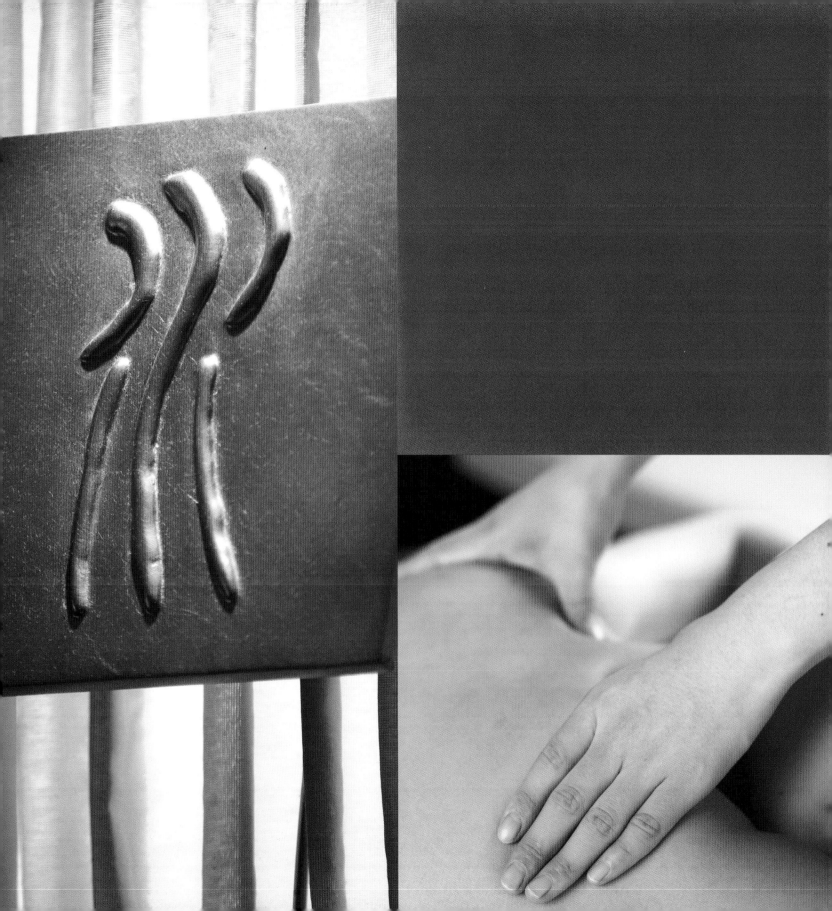

Essential Oils for Dry Skin: Sandalwood, geranium, rose, jasmine and chamomile.

Do:

⬧ Use a mild, soap-free liquid cleanser to wash face once a day.
  (In the morning just splash your face with warm water.)

⬧ Select moisturizers that delay moisture loss (like those containing
  hyaluronic acid or glycerin).

⬧ Apply moisturizer when the face is still damp to lock in the moisture.

⬧ Use sunscreen with an SPF of 15 or greater and reapply frequently
  especially when in the sun.

⬧ Use oil-based foundations to soften fine lines.

Don't:

⬧ Wash face with harsh soap.

⬧ Use grainy cleansers.

COMBINATION/SENSITIVE SKIN

Skin with an oily T-zone across the forehead and down the nose combined with a dry to normal complexion will benefit from eating predominantly cooling yin and neutral foods to rebalance the entire face. The honeysuckle facial steam (page 154) gently soothes and tones sensitive skin.

Essential Oils for Combination Skin: Sandalwood, ylang ylang, mint, coriander, camphor and cumin.

Do:

⬧ Choose cleansers specifically formulated for combination skin
  (as they are gentler on the dry areas and tougher on the oily patches).

⬧ Use a moisturizer specific for sensitive skin.

- ⊕ Use a water-based or oil-free foundation.
- ⊕ Use sunscreen with an SPF of 15 or greater and reapply frequently especially when in the sun.

Don't:

- ⊕ Use different cleansers and moisturizers for different parts of the face.

DETOXIFY YOUR SKIN

Being the body's largest organ the skin is often the first to register toxic overload—with a dull, pale and blemished appearance. While the Fourteen-Day Cleanse outlined in chapter 2 cleans the body from the inside, real skin cleaning means getting rid of all the dead cells and allowing the skin to renew and breathe more efficiently. Although skin cells are constantly being shed, body brushing (see pages 97 and 101) stimulates circulation, leaving the skin softer, cleaner and healthier. Facial steaming with two cups of boiling water, the juice of half a lemon and a dash of rosewater (or a handful of fresh petals) is a wonderful deep cleanser. Ginger- and pepper-rich foods help eliminate toxins through perspiration, while ginger and cardamom tea (recipe, page 153) is the perfect complement to a skin "detox".

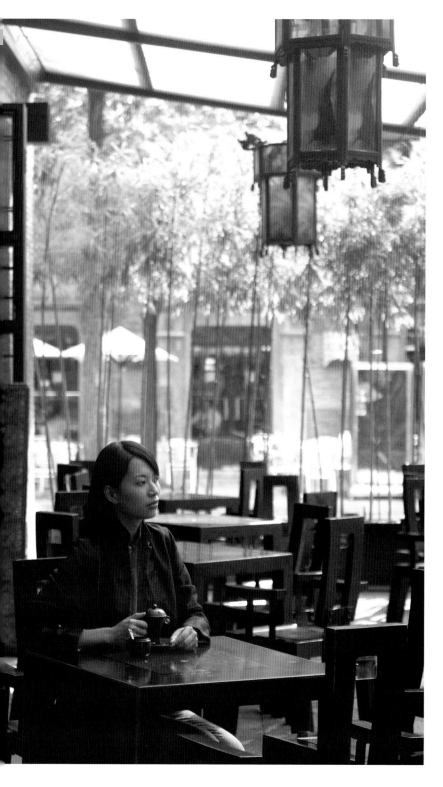

Recipes for Healthy Skin (from the inside)

Salmon Stir-Fry

(4 servings)

600-700g/20-25oz salmon steak, cut into 1cm/
    0.5-inch strips

4 cloves garlic, coarsely chopped

6-8 spring onions, cut into 2.5cm/1-inch pieces

1 piece ginger, 5cm/1.5-inches long, peeled and sliced

1 dried red chilli pepper

3 tbsp vegetable oil

1 bunch asparagus spears, cut into 2.5cm/1-inch pieces

Handful fresh spinach leaves

$^1/_2$ cup toasted almond slivers to garnish

Seasoning mix:

$^1/_4$ cup soy sauce

$^1/_2$ cup rice wine or white wine

1 tsp sugar

Combine seasoning ingredients in a glass bowl. Add salmon and toss gently. Leave to marinate for a least one hour. Drain fish and reserve half the marinade. Heat oil in pan. Add half of the garlic, spring onions, ginger and pepper and stir quickly. Add salmon and cook for two to three minutes. Add remaining garlic, spring onions, ginger, pepper, asparagus and spinach. Stir-fry for a further two to three minutes until fish and vegetables are cooked. Garnish with almond slivers and serve over rice if desired.

Honeysuckle Blossom Tea

(4 servings)

2 tbsp fresh or 1 tbsp dried honeysuckle flowers

$^1/_2$ litre (1 pint) boiling water

Put flowers in a teapot and pour in boiling water.

Cover and steep for at least 10 minutes before drinking.

Cardamom and Ginger Tea

(4 servings)

2 tsp cardamom shavings

2 tsp ginger root shavings

$^1/_2$ litre (1 pint) boiling water

Honey to taste

Mix shavings of cardamom and ginger root in a cup
with boiling water. Allow to steep. Add honey to taste.
Drink 2-3 cups per day.

Raspberry Smoothie

(1 serving)

100g/3.5oz raspberries (or strawberries), fresh or frozen

1 small banana, peeled

1 small pot of yoghurt with active bacterial cultures

150ml soya milk

Blend all ingredients until completely mixed
and serve in a glass.

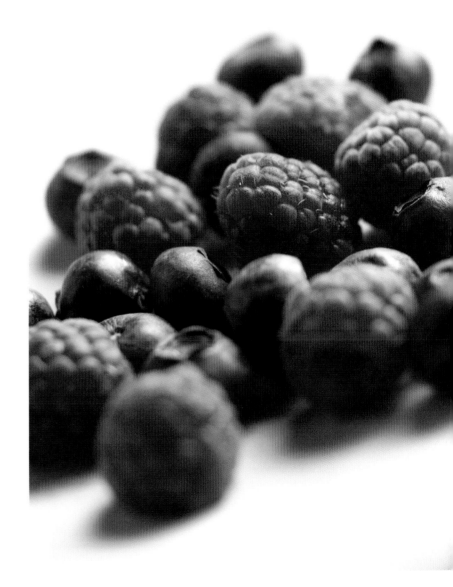

Recipes for Healthy Skin (from the outside)

Honeysuckle Facial Steam

(*makes one treatment*)

$1/4$ cup dried honeysuckle flowers or 4 honeysuckle tea bags

2 cups water

Bring water to the boil. Put the honeysuckle flowers or tea bags in a bowl and pour the water over them. Steep for 2 minutes covered with a small towel. To steam the face simply place the bowl on a solid surface. Remove towel and place over your head. Lean over the bowl and let the vapours hydrate your skin for up to 10 minutes. Pat face dry with a soft, dry towel.

Walnut Yoghurt Scrub

(*makes one treatment*)

Packed with essential oils, walnuts lubricate the skin without clogging.

$1/4$ cup finely chopped walnuts

$1/4$ cup plain yoghurt

Blend the walnuts and yoghurt together. Wet the face and rub the blend gently into the skin to cleanse and exfoliate, avoiding the delicate tissue around the eye. Rinse with tepid water and dry the face with a soft towel. Use 1-2 times a week to keep skin clean, healthy and radiant.

Honey Apricot Mask

(*makes one treatment*)

A neutral mask that softens and hydrates the skin—for face and body.

$1/2$ cup honey

2 apricots, peeled and coarsely chopped

Mix honey and apricots together in a bowl. Apply to face and neck, massaging gently with fingertips. Leave for 10 minutes before removing with warm water. Pat skin dry with a soft towel. If using as a body treatment, apply all over while sitting in the bath. Leave for 10 minutes and rinse under the shower.

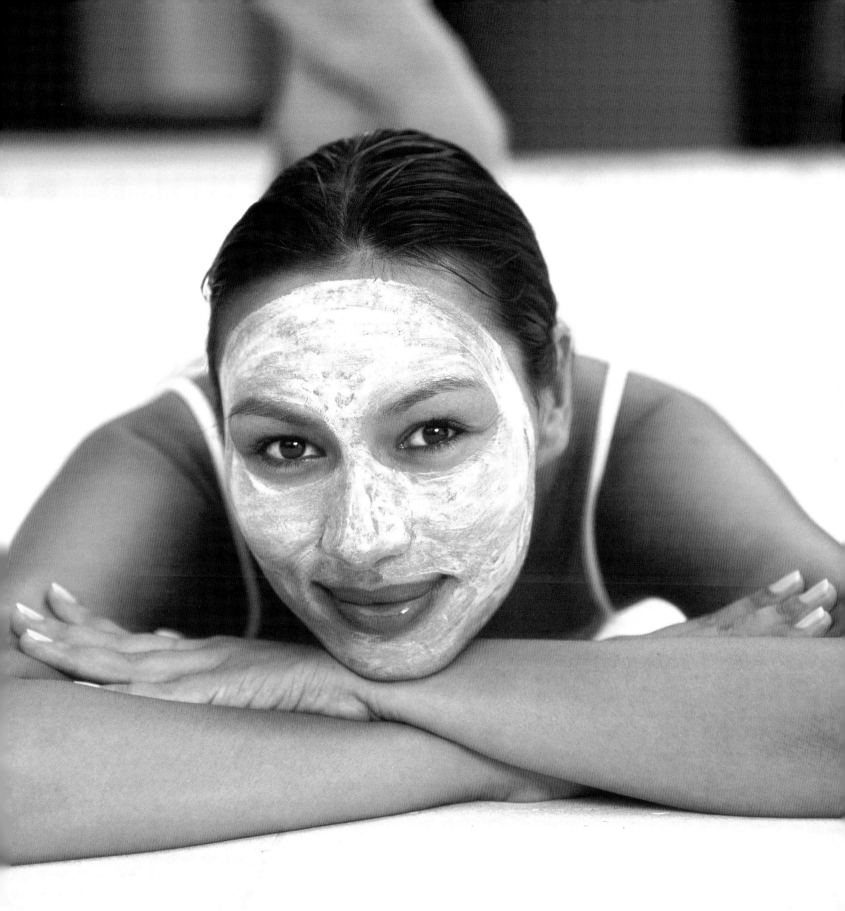

Qi for Beautiful Hair

"Shining . . . hair on a woman is called 'Cloud-hair' and is admired . . . especially when the growth of hair is also strong and luxuriant. In any description of a beautiful woman, her hair is usually the first thing to be mentioned."

—Wolfram Eberhard, *A Dictionary of Chinese Symbols* (1986)

To the Chinese hair that is anything but strong, healthy and shiny is indicative of kidney *Qi* imbalance. By simply examining the texture of hair you can get an insight into a person's overall health and harmony. For example, dry and brittle hair is seen as evidence of yin deficiency and "heat" in the blood.

Concurrent with the female body developing around a seven-year cycle, hair is at its strongest during the twenties when kidney *Qi* refinement occurs and women are at their most fertile. By 49 years or so with kidney *Qi* waning, hair becomes weaker and more prone to greying and falling out. "Grey" hair is really a combination of normally pigmented hair interspersed with white. Hair turns white when the pigment cells at the base of the hair follicle stop being produced, a result of either genetics or lifestyle factors like inadequate diet, cigarette smoking and stress.

While hair type and volume is genetic, overall hair condition is personal. Crash diets and high fat, processed foods are detrimental to hair health while medications like the oral contraceptive, diet pills, sleeping tablets and even some cold remedies can make hair dull, brittle and lifeless.

Although specific hair products and treatments will improve texture and condition, the key to maintaining a healthy head of hair is ensuring the roots and follicles are well nourished from within. This means regulating the body's internal environment and improving circulation to the scalp so that nutrients and *Qi* can nourish the follicles.

EATING WITH THE SEASONS

To keep hair healthy, shiny and really strong, nature's rhythms must be matched by eating with the seasons as outlined in chapter 2. In addition, the following foods and herbs add lustre and shine to hair.

Fruits and Nuts: Blackberries, chestnuts, Chinese red and black dates, grapes, papayas, plums, tangerines and walnuts.

Vegetables: Black soya beans (reputed to make Asian hair lustrous and black), yellow soya beans, carrots, celery, chives, fennel, green leafy vegetables like spinach, cabbage and *bak choi*, onions, parsnips, pumpkins, red beans, arame seaweed, sweet potatoes and squash.

Grains and Seeds: Black sesame seeds, oats, sweet rice, brown rice, whole wheat and pumpkin seeds.

Proteins: Lean meat, fish, chicken, eggs and kidneys.

Herbs: Chinese parsley, cinnamon, cloves, *dang gui*, ginger, licorice root, safflower and wolfberry (which provides excellent protection against premature greying and hair fall).

Water: Taken either as cooling drinks or for heat and warmth, daily fluid is essential for a healthy head of hair.

Recommended Chinese herbal formulations:

Royal Jelly and Ginseng Formula (Jinnao Yang Seng Wan Jaing) from Tong Ren Tang.
Dosage: One or two capsules daily with food.

H4H Hair Formula from Eu Yan Sang (only available in Hong Kong).
Dosage: As recommended by a Chinese medicine practitioner.

HAIR CARE FOR THE SEASONS
SPRING

After the cooler winter months, hair will benefit from a new colour or style. The Fourteen Day Spring Cleanse outlined in chapter 2 is a great hair "detox", cleaning from within and nourishing the roots in preparation for the summer months ahead. To regain lost vitality in the hair and scalp, try the following Spring Revitalizer.

Spring Revitalizer: Mix equal quantities of zinc oxide cream (the cream oil-in-water

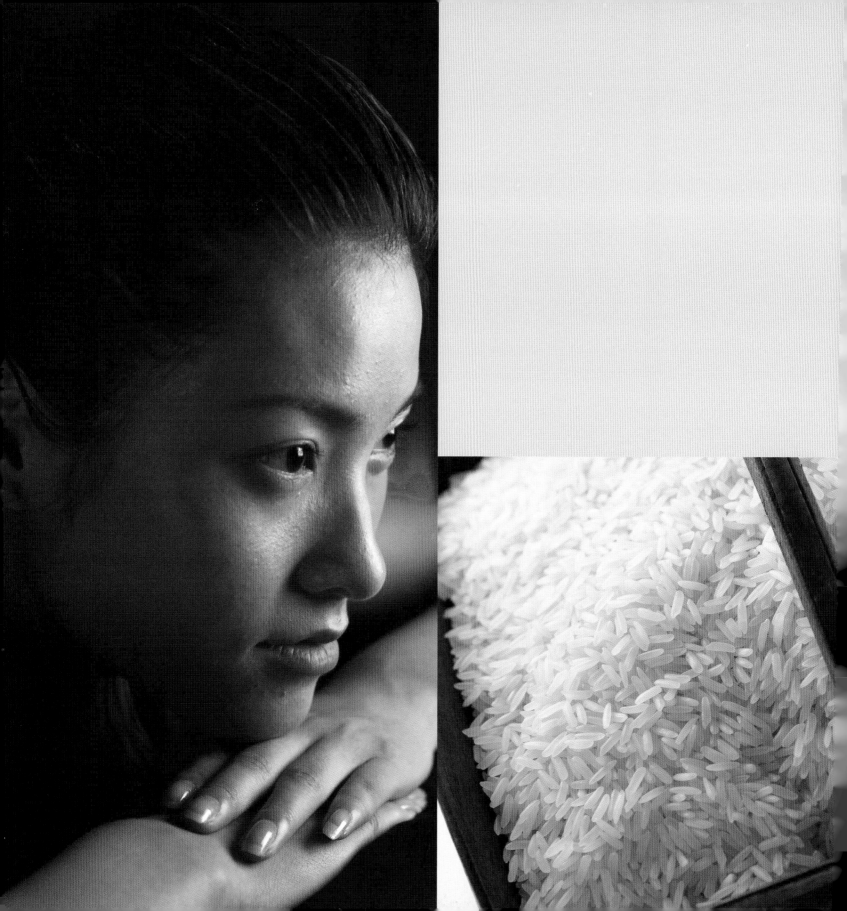

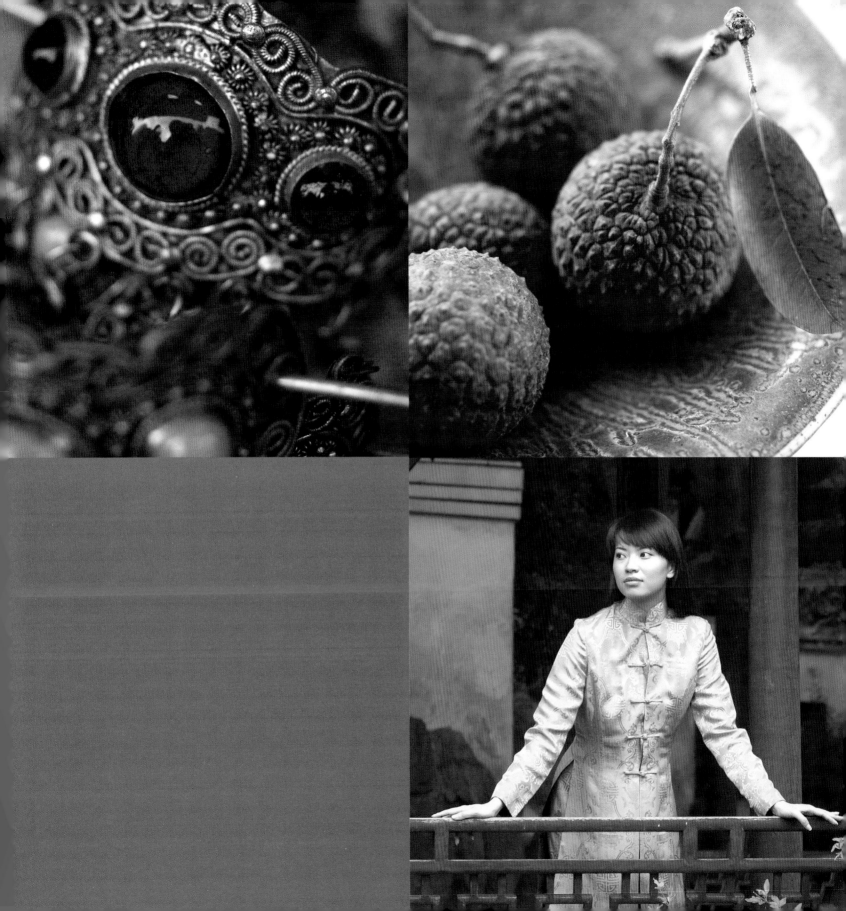

emulsion available in chemists) with regular mouthwash and two large sprigs of crushed fresh mint until the mixture is quite runny. Apply to the scalp in 2.5cm (1 inch) partings and massage gently for about five minutes. Wrap head in cling film and warm, wet towels for about 15 minutes, changing the towels as they cool. Wash and condition as normal. If hair is particularly dry and lacklustre, use a heavy moisturizing conditioner after massaging with the zinc cream. Spread evenly through the hair and wrap in a warm damp towel for 15 minutes. Rinse thoroughly and shampoo and condition as normal. Although time consuming, when applied twice weekly for a few weeks the results can be incredible.

SUMMER

The sun's rays can burn hair, weakening its protein structure and reducing its elasticity (so it breaks more easily). Combined with chlorine and salt water this can spell disaster. Just as the skin should be protected from the sun so too should hair. Sun protection sprays and leave-in conditioners must be applied to hair regularly exposed to the sun.

Summer Hair Protection: To protect hair when swimming, mix some waterproof high-factor sunscreen oil with a thick leave-in conditioner and apply it in sections along the length of the hair. Comb through for even distribution. The oil and conditioner combination protects hair from chlorine and sea salt while also conditioning and maintaining moisture. For best results reapply after swimming.

Summer Deep-Conditioning Treatment: A weekly pre-shampoo deep conditioner nourishes and moisturizes the hair from the roots keeping it healthy and shiny all summer long. Whisk together two eggs, two half eggshells of olive oil (or light vegetable oil), half a ripe avocado and 50ml of purified water. Work mixture into the hair with fingertips and leave for 10 minutes before shampooing as normal.

LONG SUMMER

Characterized by summer rain and humidity hair is prone to becoming frizzy during the Long Summer season with curly fine hair being especially vulnerable. No matter how it is

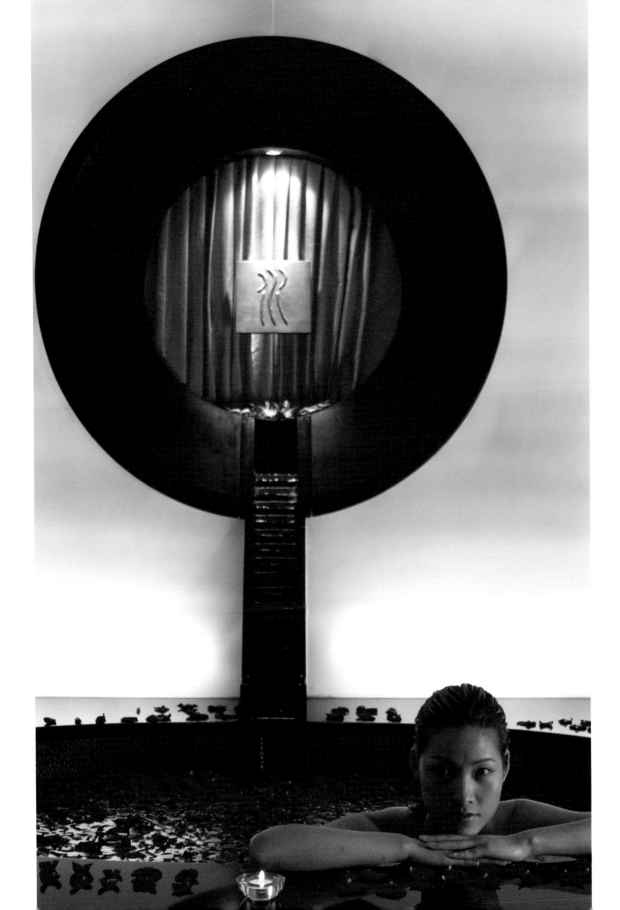

styled, once exposed to humidity, it reverts to its natural configuration. To protect hair from becoming frizzy use silicone-containing products that discourage moisture absorption into the hair shaft. These products are water resistant and generally wash out easily. However, a little is enough as if overused they leave the hair brittle and dull.

AUTUMN

After the heat of summer, dry, dull and split hair can be the norm in autumn. Split ends must be trimmed and moisturized.

Autumn Home Hair Therapy: To help regain hair's natural elasticity, mix together 60g/2.4oz of soft margarine, 30g/1.2oz of butter, 90g/3.6oz of single cream and 90g/3.6oz of heavy conditioner. Whisk in a blender and apply to the hair in sections, working in well with the fingers. Cover hair with a warm damp towel and leave for a minimum of 15 minutes or overnight under a shower cap and towel. Rinse thoroughly and shampoo as normal. Reapply frequently until hair looks and feels healthy, shiny and strong.

WINTER

Winter is the worst time for flaky and itchy scalps. In colder climates heavier winter clothing can also make the scalp sweat and the hair frizzy. Daily shampooing and conditioning is essential as less frequent washing exacerbates flakiness and makes hair limp.

Itchy Scalp Tonic: Shake together equal quantities of witch hazel and regular mouthwash (60ml each). Add 15ml of vodka, shake, and apply to the scalp, parting hair and using cotton wool. Massage the scalp for five minutes to promote a balanced *Qi* before shampooing as normal. The scalp will feel soothed and refreshed.

NOURISH YOUR HAIR

✣ **Daily shampooing and conditioning adds moisture and shine while also exercising the scalp muscles and encouraging faster and healthier growth.**

- Wear a hat or scarf to protect the hair in extreme weather conditions.
- If living in a warm climate or swimming regularly use a weekly pre-shampoo deep conditioner to protect your hair.
- Guard against split ends by avoiding overbrushing.
- Brush hair gently with a blunt saw-cut comb or a brush with long, widely spaced, plastic bristles.
- Wash hairbrush and comb weekly by soaking in water with a few drops of tea tree essential oil.
- If wearing hair tied back, do not pull it too hard. Spread a little conditioner around the fabric of the tie or elastic to further protect the hair.
- Caffeine (in coffee, certain teas and soft drinks) dehydrates the hair so is best reduced or avoided altogether.

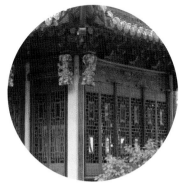

Qi for Beautiful Hands, Feet and Nails

"If a woman has fine slender fingers, these are compared to onion shoots, and in order to make them even more attractive they are coloured with sap . . . The long fingernails affected until quite recently by rich Chinese were regarded as a symbol of wealth. Nail guards to prevent accidental breakage of these status symbols were in use from the seventh century AD onwards."

—Wolfram Eberhard, *A Dictionary of Chinese Symbols (1986)*

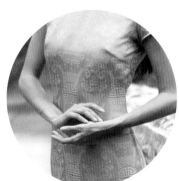

In Chinese thinking, the hands and feet are mirrors of the body and share reflex points corresponding with body organs. For example, the inside foot from the big toe to the heel represents the spine and pressure applied to the reflex points in this area can relieve backache, headache, stomach ulcers and a host of other stress-related conditions. Foot reflexology is discussed in chapter 3 while traditional Chinese palmistry is covered below.

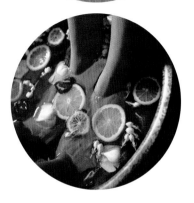

TRADITIONAL CHINESE PALMISTRY

The study of the surface of the hands and wrists is a deeply rooted diagnostic tool in TCM. The hand is readily available and can be examined painlessly, relatively quickly and without expensive diagnostic machinery.

Just as reflexology maps the body through the feet, palmistry does so with the hands. Combining age-old wisdom with modern scientific interpretation has led to a deeper understanding of the relationship between the appearance and lines on the hand and disease prevention. While not a complete medical diagnostic system in itself, when used as part of an overall health assessment, Chinese medical palmistry reveals useful information about the workings of the body (physical and emotional) and possible constitutional predispositions.

The Five Phase System of Chinese palmistry (influenced by Buddhism) is the most popular today. This maintains that the appearance of the hands can reveal the *san hou* or three periods in a person's life: their past (*xian zhen*), their present (*zi zhen*) and their future (*lai zhen*).

During a typical examination the physician will examine the shape of the hands, their look, colour, thickness and relative moisture as well as the fingernails and lines on the palms (*shou xian*) to determine a person's strengths and diagnose any potential disease. Hot hands with dry, scaly or red skin are symptomatic of excess internal heat which must be quelled with cooling foods and drinks, while cold and pale hands are a sign of cold and stagnant *Qi* that needs replenishing with hot, yang energy. *Dang gui* and Chinese licorice separately or mixed together and drunk as a tea are perfect for revitalizing yang *Qi*.

Each of the five fingers reflects a person's health at different stages in their life: the thumb, childhood; index finger, youth; middle finger, adulthood; ring finger, later adult life and the little finger, health in old age. When all five fingers are strong with good development and the fingertips are red or ruddy this is a sign of healthy blood and *Qi* circulation.

FINGERNAILS

Ruled by the liver, a healthy nail should be strong but flexible, smooth and pale red in colour. If the nail's colour, appearance or strength is any different, there is thought to be disharmony in the system (e.g. thin and brittle nails are a sign of *Qi* and blood deficiency).

Each part of the nail is significant and related to the viscera and organs in the body: the thumb pertains to the lungs; index finger to the large intestine; middle finger, the pericardium; ring finger, the internal membrane; inner side of the small finger, the heart; and its outer side, the small intestine.

LUNULAE

The crescent shapes at the base of each nail are called the lunulae or "health circle" and are believed to reflect a person's general physical health (especially cardiovascular). Lunulae tend to follow from parent to child which in TCM is a good indication of "one's former heaven".

Well-proportioned lunulae on each finger (with the largest and most obvious being on the thumb and getting a little smaller with each successive finger) is a sign of health and bal-

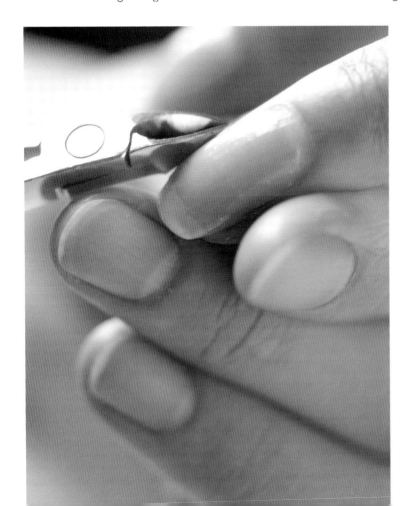

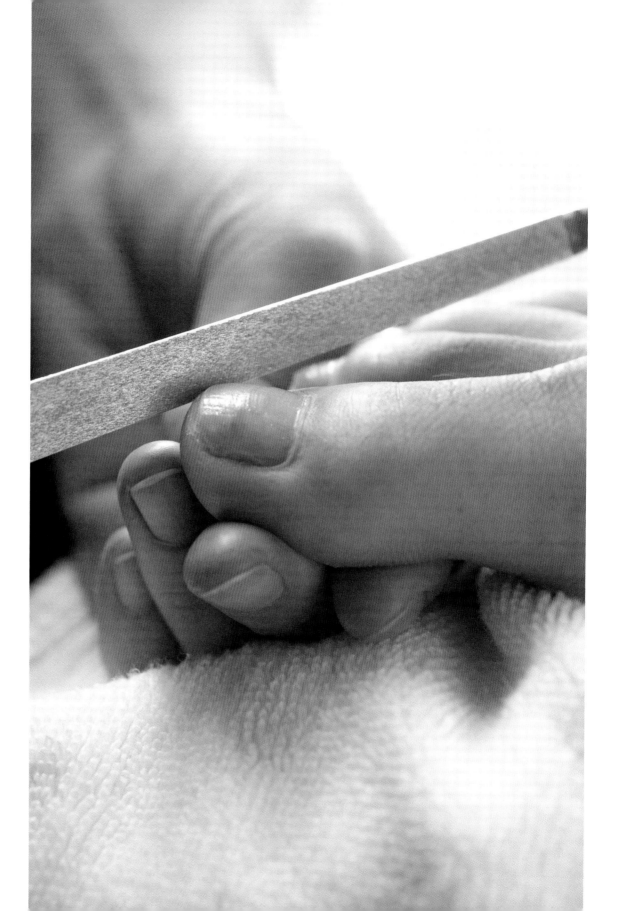

ance. Those with smaller and fewer lunulae are thought to have weakened physical strength and need more warming yang foods and spices, while people with larger and disproportionate lunulae have excess yang and need the yin energy of cooling foods and drinks.

As nails are less porous and less absorbent than skin they lose moisture a lot faster so daily massage with moisturizing cream or petroleum jelly is essential to stimulate circulation, and rehydrate and strengthen the nail bed.

FEEDING THE HANDS, FEET AND NAILS

While manicures and pedicures help nails look better, to keep them at their best they need nurturing from within. Recommended foods are listed below. As the nail is about 16% water, adequate daily fluid intake is essential for sturdy, strong nails.

Fruits, Nuts and Seeds: Blackberries, chestnuts, Chinese red and black dates, papaya, peaches, pears, pumpkin, red grapes, strawberries, tangerines, walnuts, sesame seeds and flaxseeds.

Vegetables: Asparagus, soya beans, green leafy vegetables like spinach, cabbage and *bak choi*, broccoli, carrots, celery, chives, fennel, green and red beans, kale, mushrooms, onions, parsnips, red peppers, snow peas, tomatoes, watercress, squash and shallots.

Herbs and Spices: Chinese licorice root, Chinese parsley (coriander), chives, cinnamon, cloves, *dang gui*, garlic, ginger, ginseng, wheat grass and gingko biloba.

Other Foods: Lean meats, eggs, chicken, lamb, pork, oysters, oily fish (especially those with fine bones like sardines and herrings) and dairy products.

Recommended Chinese herbal formulations:

Australian Natural Deer Velvet Powder Capsules (Lu Rong Jiao Nang) from Tong Ren Tang.
Dosage: Four capsules a day.

Royal Jelly and Ginseng Formula (Jinnao Yang Seng Wan Jaing) from Tong Ren Tang.
Dosage: One or two capsules daily with food.

Ten Nourishing Herbs (Shi Quan Da Bu Wan) from Tong Ren Tang.
Dosage: 30 pills, twice a day.

TO MAINTAIN BEAUTIFUL HANDS AND NAILS

- Always wear gloves when doing work in the home.
- Rub white iodine on nails with cotton wool to make them stronger (regular iodine will stain).
- Gently erase calluses and rough edges on heels and soles with a damp pumice stone after a bath or shower.
- Allow the feet to breathe naturally by going barefoot.
- Enjoy a manicure and pedicure as often as possible.

Recipe for Healthy Hands and Feet (from the outside)

Ginger and Chinese Licorice Hand and Foot Soak

(makes one treatment)

Ginger stimulates the circulation bringing energy and *Qi* to the hands and feet, while Chinese licorice protects nails and feet.

200-300g (9-12oz) ginger, cut into long strips

6-8 slices of Chinese licorice root

6 cups water

Pound ginger with a mallet to break the fibres. Lightly pound the licorice root to release its essence. Boil ginger and licorice with water in a glass or enamel saucepan for five to 10 minutes until the liquid resembles weak tea. Strain, reserving liquid and cool slightly. Soak hands and/or feet in the solution for 10-15 minutes until water is tepid before drying with a soft towel.

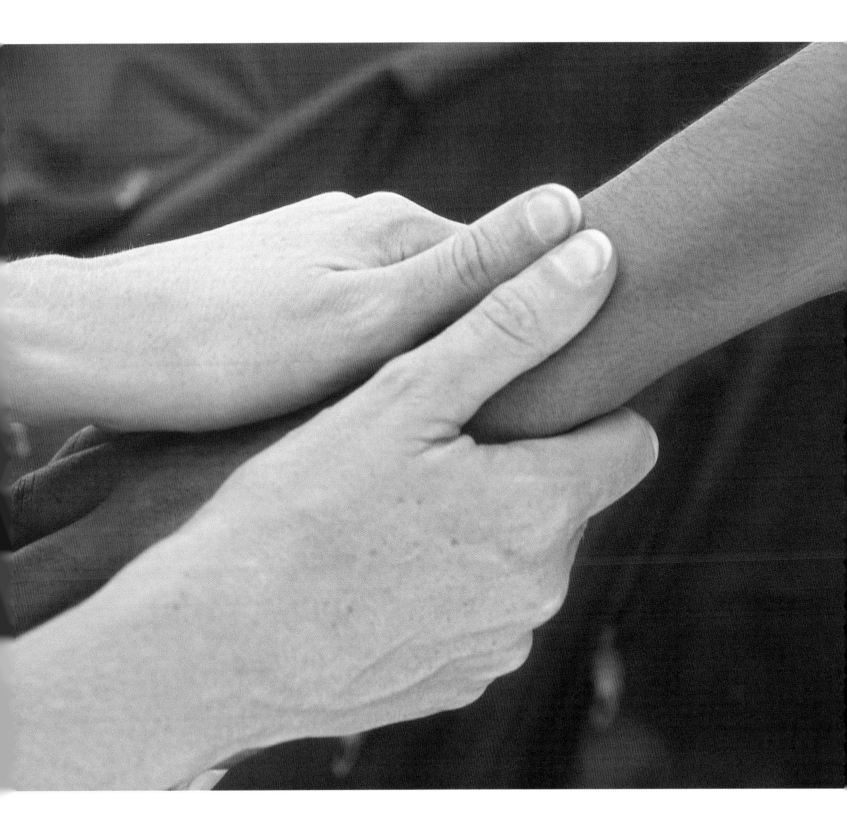

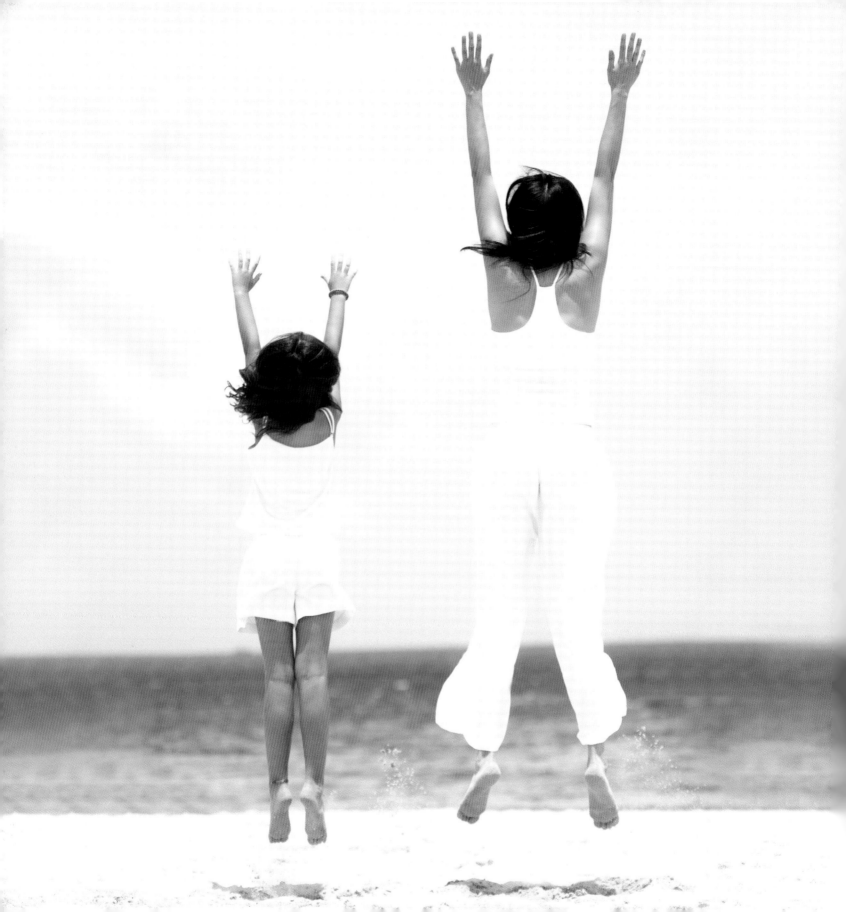

CHAPTER 6

Vitality, Chinese-style:
energy, immunity and sleep

"When the mind is calm and stable, the vitality of life circulates harmoniously throughout the body. If the body is nourished and protected by this circulation of vitality, how can it possibly become ill?"

—*Yellow Emperor's Classic of Internal Medicine* (220BC)

Qi for Energy

"Health, wellbeing and long life can only be achieved by guarding
    against squandering one's *Qi,*
Using breath and movement to maintain the free flow of *Qi* and blood,
Aligning with the natural forces of the seasons
and cultivating the tranquil heart and mind."

— *Yellow Emperor's Classic of Internal Medicine* (220BC)

In Chinese the word "vitality" is used to signify a combination of energy, spirit and the vital essence of life that is the basis of health and longevity and the foundation of immunity and resistance.

We spend time, money and energy itself in the quest for energy. "Tired all the time" ("TATT") is one of the commonest reasons people consult their doctor. Poor diet, inadequate exercise, lack of sleep, pollution, hormones and emotional stress are just some of the causes of reduced energy.

If skipping meals, eating on the run and processed and refined foods constitute your weekly diet, the chances are that you are not getting the fuel you need to keep energy circulating harmoniously and your body working at its best. Energy-boosting tips are outlined below; ways of eating in harmony with nature's cycles are covered in chapter 2.

Chinese medicine also looks beyond the physical to find an emotional explanation for energy imbalances in the system. This is especially relevant for the management of excessive anger and many stress-related conditions which are a leading cause of reduced energy and immunity and a subsequent internal *Qi* crisis. The breathing exercises described here are especially relevant for conserving and increasing the body's energy.

DEEP BREATHING FOR ENERGY

To the ancient Chinese, breathing is energy. The word *Qi* refers to breath and both words share the same Chinese character. The regulation of the breath is a common feature of Chinese movement therapies such as *qi gung* and *tai chi*.

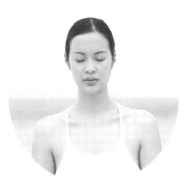

Correctly performed, deep breathing exercises encourage the body to breathe from within, expelling waste completely, slowing the heart rate and stabilizing blood pressure. Just 10 to 15 minutes of deep breathing each day either at home or in the office can reap enormous long-term health benefits by improving the circulation of *Qi* and boosting the body's innate energy.

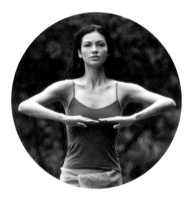

There are four distinct stages to correct deep breathing practice: inhalation, retention, exhalation and pause. It is imperative that each stage flows smoothly to the next. Begin by either sitting or lying with the stomach relaxed, shoulders loose and spine erect. Empty the lungs completely with a forced exhalation and a strong contraction of the abdominal wall.

Inhalation: Let the stomach relax and start inhaling slowly through the nostrils for a count of six to eight seconds, drawing the breath deep down into the bottom of the lungs so the stomach expands like a balloon. When the base of the lungs are full, continue inhaling smoothly through the ribcage to the top of the lungs. It is not necessary to fill the lungs completely with each inhalation and never force the breath.

Retention: Hold the breath for six to eight seconds by tucking the chin in slightly to "lock" the throat.

Exhalation: Relax the chin before slowly starting to exhale through the nose, keeping the tongue pressed to the roof of the mouth. Starting at the top of the lungs, gradually increase the force of exhalation until a strong and steady flow is established. At the end of the exhalation pull the entire abdominal area inwards to push the diaphragm into the chest thereby expelling any residual stale air.

Pause: When the lungs are completely empty, tuck the chin in towards the body to close the throat. Pause for a few seconds to relax the abdominal area before slowly starting the next inhalation.

Continue this sequence for 10-15 minutes. If the breath tends to burst out in explosive gusts, it has been retained for too long. Try a shorter retention. It is not the duration or volume of breath retained that is important, but the smooth, rhythmic regularity of the entire breathing process.

EATING FOR ENERGY

A natural reaction to waning energy levels is to load the body with sugars and refined carbohydrates that give a rapid surge of energy. This is quickly followed by burnout, which over time leads to chronic fatigue, poor digestion and sleep disturbances. A fresh, seasonal diet packed with unprocessed grains, green vegetables, lean meats and fruits ensures your body gets what it needs to keep energy levels soaring. In addition, a Chinese practitioner would prescribe herbs such as ginseng (*Radix panax ginseng*), Chinese or Korean ginseng, Siberian ginseng (*Radix elutherococcus senticosus*) or huang qi (*Radix astragali membranacei*).

ENERGY BOOSTERS

✦ **Eat with the seasons.**

✦ **Start each day with an energy-packed power breakfast.**

✦ **Eat regularly through the day to keep blood sugar levels evenly balanced.**

✦ **Cut down or avoid stimulants like coffee and caffeinated drinks.**

✦ **Eat more lean protein-rich foods like lean meat, chicken, fish and pulse vegetables.**

✦ **Cut processed and refined foods.**

✦ **Follow the "75 per cent" rule (see page 51).**

✦ **Avoid heavy meals (especially late at night).**

- Eat a variety of foods of various flavours, energies and actions.

- Listen to your body and respond accordingly.

- Sunrise (yang) is the most active part of the day. Make the most of this by rising earlier or keeping curtains open to catch the early morning sun.

- Stop smoking: filling the lungs with smoke diminishes *Qi*.

- Move: yoga and other Asian exercises enhance the circulation of *Qi* through the body.

- Enjoy energizing massage therapies especially during times of increased stress and exhaustion (see chapter 3).

Recommended Chinese herbal formulations:

Black Chicken, White Phoenix Pills (Wuchi Paifeng Wan) from Plum Flower Brand. These come in boxes of 10 wax "eggs" each containing small uncoated pills.

Dosage: Crack off wax and take half the contents twice daily, swallowed with, or dissolved in, water.

Australian Natural Deer Velvet Powdered Capsules (Lu Rong Jiao Nang) from Tong Ren Tang.

Dosage: 30 pills, twice a day.

Blood Tonic Formula (Bu Zhen Pills) from Eu Yan Sang.

Dosage: As recommended by a Chinese medicine practitioner.

Recommended supplements (follow manufacturer's dosage instructions):

- Multivitamin and mineral complex.

- B Complex vitamins.

- Essential Fatty Acids (EFAs) or flaxseed oil.

Recipes for Boosting Energy

Energizing Bean Soup

(*2 servings*)

An ancient Chinese recipe adapted to Western tastes
that is especially beneficial for treating chronic tiredness.
Follow this basic recipe and adapt for taste.

2 tsp sesame oil

1 cup small white beans

$^1/_2$ cup small red beans

5 cloves garlic, chopped

1 stalk celery

1 large carrot, diced

$^1/_2$ tsp sugar

Pinch of salt

Soak beans overnight in water. Dry chestnuts and black
beans can also be added. Heat oil in a preheated wok or
heavy skillet until it starts to smoke. Add the chopped garlic
and a pinch of salt, followed by the beans, and sauté until
tender. Add sugar, celery and carrot and cook until the
mixture begins to sweat. Add enough water to cover and
bring to the boil, stirring well. Reduce heat, cover and simmer for about two hours (adding more water if needed).

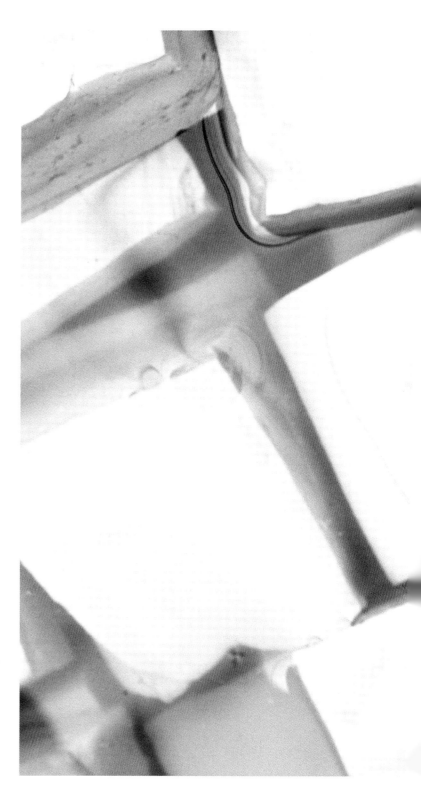

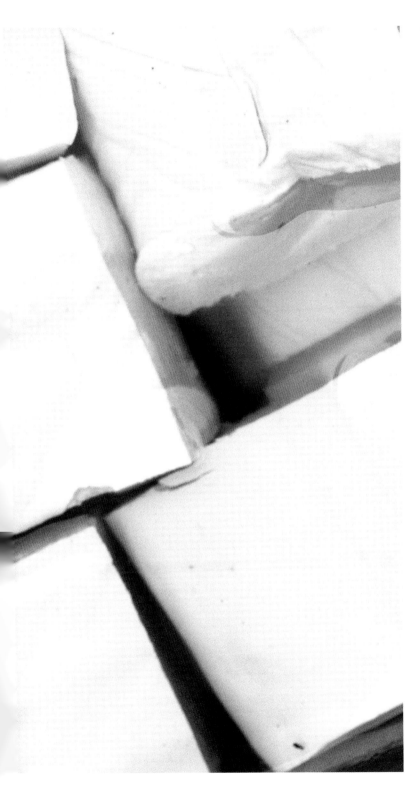

When almost cooked, season to taste. Chopped or tinned tomatoes can be added if desired. Keep refrigerated and eat daily for breakfast or lunch for three to four weeks.

Steamed Beancurd Roll with Fresh Ginger

(4-6 servings)

60g/2.4oz fresh ginseng

1 beancurd roll

1 slice ginger

A few red dates

Water or vegetable stock

Soak red dates in water until tender. Remove seeds and rinse and drain. Rinse and drain the beancurd roll and fresh ginger. Cut beancurd into large pieces and put all ingredients into a large pot to steam. Add water or vegetable stock until nearly full. Cover and steam over high heat for 1 1/2 hours. Season with salt and serve.

Qi for Immunity

"When the spleen and pancreas are full of energy, the body will be immune from disease."

—*Zhang Zhong Jing* (300AD)

Comprising the spleen, lymph nodes, thymus, tonsils, bone and white blood cells, the immune system fights off enemies (such as bacteria, viruses and cancer-causing free radicals) and repairs any damage they cause.

In Chinese medicine "health" implies the ability to correct any potential imbalances occurring in the body before they actually arise. A strong immune system is a fundamental part of this. Immune function can be either in deficiency or excess; neither is ideal. If the body's defense system is weakened through inadequate diet, fatigue or illness, an invading pathogen can easily initiate a strong reaction within, producing symptoms like fever, chills, pains and aches. Conversely, as evident in certain cases of irritable bowel syndrome, asthma and psoriasis, among other conditions, the body's immunity can become excessive and sensitized, initiating a self-imposed reaction to itself. Treatment in both cases rests on rebalancing immunity so it is once again strong and in control.

With the onset of seasonal change, the body becomes more vulnerable to infection. To keep immune function working optimally through the year we must work with nature by eating with the seasons (as outlined in chapter 2). Acupuncture, massage, herbs and tonics further balance the body's internal environment, keeping the immune system well nourished and balanced.

For boosting immunity naturally, think green. Packed with antioxidant goodness, fresh greens are possibly the best investment for immune protection. In summer, choose salad greens, broccoli and spinach juiced and at meals. Cabbage, brussel sprouts, *bak choi* and other Chinese greens are ideal for winter.

Spirulina, a type of blue-green freshwater algae packed with vitamins and minerals, is a noted immune enhancer. Available from good health food shops, it can be added to juices starting with one teaspoon per day and slowly increasing to two to three teaspoons.

Scientific experiments on Chinese herbs such as *bai zhu (Rhizoma atractylodis macrocephalae)*, *huang qi (Radix astragali)* and *ling zhi (Ganoderma lucidum)* have shown that their use can enhance and/or regulate immune function.

A positive outlook on life has also been shown to contribute to a healthy immune system.

Recommended Chinese herbal formulations:

Jade Screen Teapills (Yu Ping Feng San Wan) from Plum Flower Brand.

Traditionally used for common colds and allergies.

Dosage: Eight pills, three times daily (can be increased to 12 pills, three times a day, if needed).

Australian Natural Deer Velvet Powder Capsules (Lu Rong Jiao Nang) from Tong Ren Tang.

Dosage: Four capsules a day.

Royal Jelly and Ginseng Formula (Jinnao Yang Seng Wan Jaing) from Tong Ren Tang.

Dosage: 30 pills, twice daily.

Lingzhi Cracked Spores Powder Capsules from Eu Yan Sang.

Dosage: As recommended by a Chinese medicine practitioner.

Recommended supplements (follow manufacturer's dosage instructions):
- ❖ **Probiotic supplements.**
- ❖ **Antioxidant vitamins A, C, and E.**
- ❖ **Zinc and selenium.**

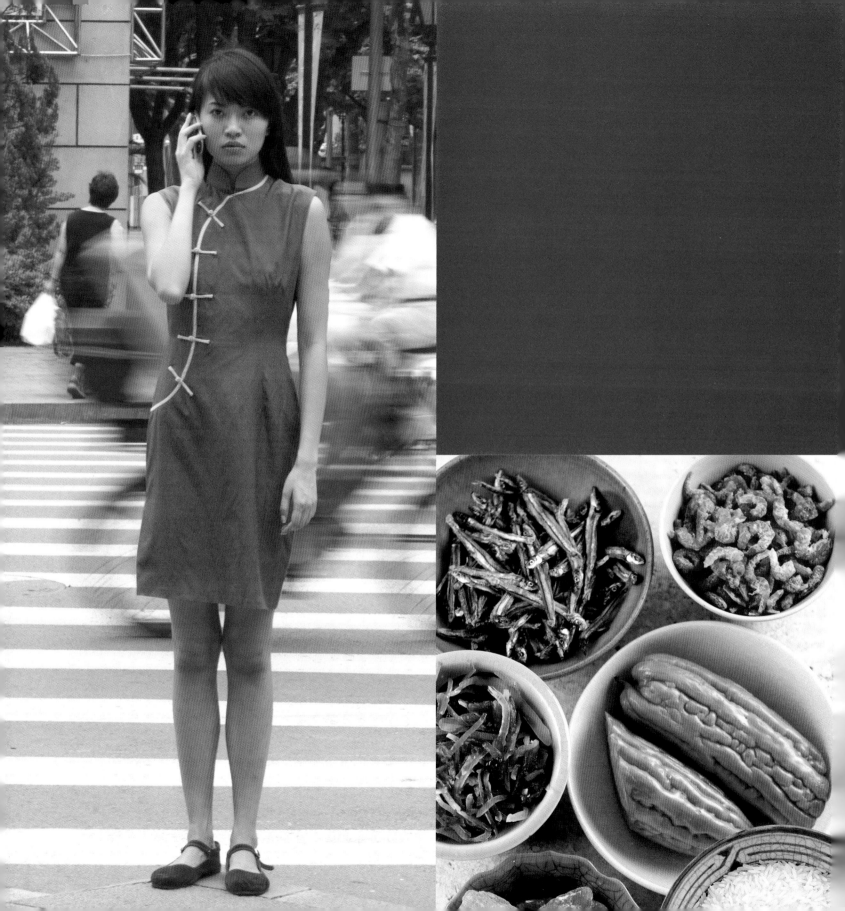

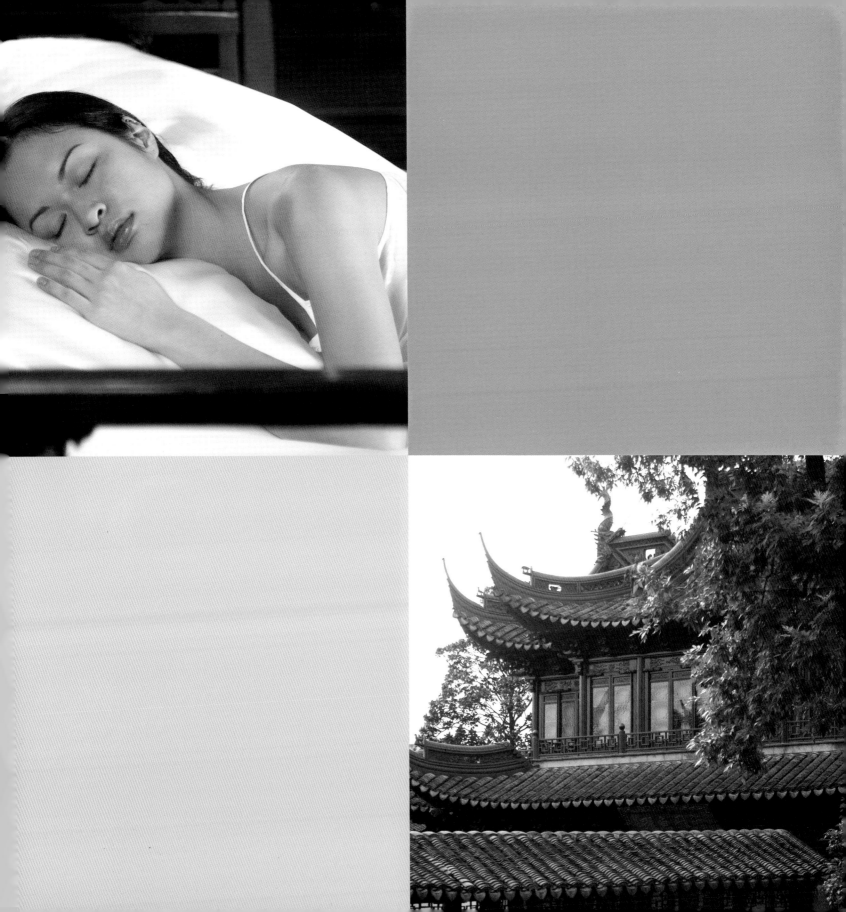

Recipes for Increasing Immunity
BOOSTER JUICES

SPRING

Dandelion Tonic: page 65.

Spring Cocktail

(*1 serving*)

¹/₂ a small papaya, peeled and deseeded

1 orange, peeled

Juice of 1 lime

Juice fruits together and pour into a long glass. If consistency is a little thick top with sparkling water. To make into a delicious spring smoothie, blend with two tablespoons of low fat yoghurt with active bacterial cultures.

SUMMER

Summer Mint Magic

(*1 serving*)

1 small pineapple

1 apple

Handful mint leaves

Remove the skin from the pineapple and cut into chunks. Juice ingredients and pour into a tall glass.

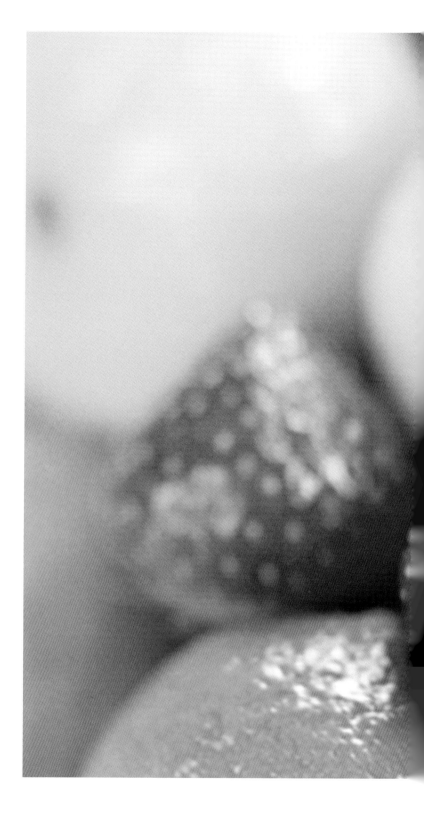

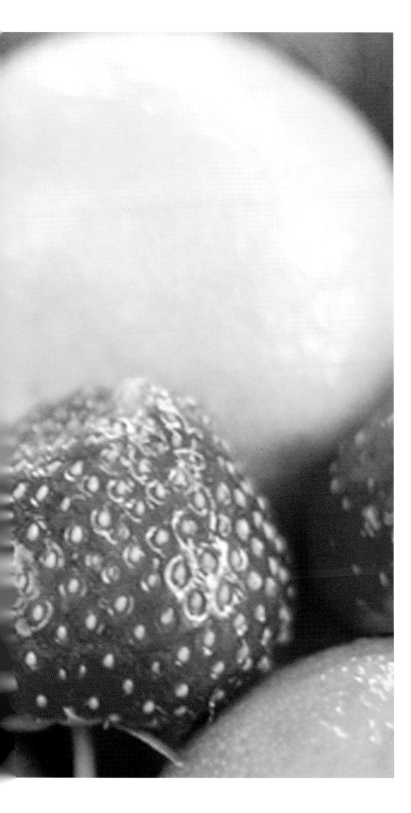

Cooling Peppermint Tea

(2 servings)

Peppermint cleanses the breath, reduces body odour, cools you down and is stimulating.

25g/1 oz peppermint

A few slices of lemon

2 cups water

Add peppermint to a teapot of boiling water. Top with a few slices of lemon and let it steep, covered, for about 10 minutes. Drink.

LONG SUMMER

Beetroot Bliss

(2 servings)

2 whole green apples

1 ¹/₂ large beetroot

1 stick celery

1 fingernail-size knob of ginger

Wash all ingredients and put in the juicer.

Garnish with a slice of apple and drink.

AUTUMN

Pear Cocktail

(4-6 servings)

3 pears

1 large carrot

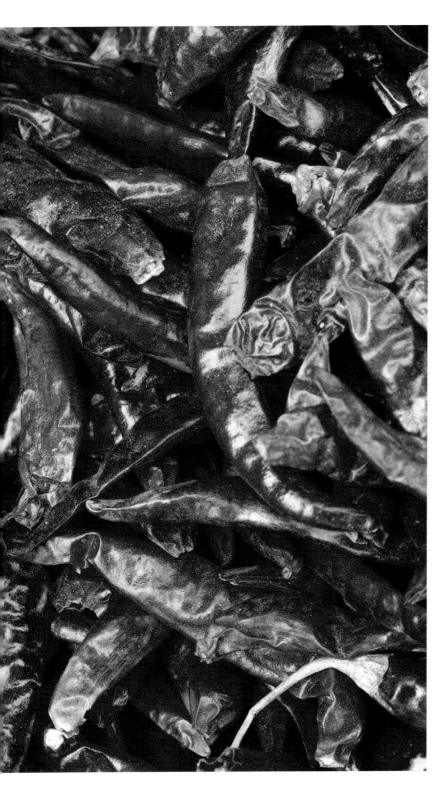

10 apricot kernels

Rock sugar (to taste)

1 ½ litres of water

Boil ingredients together for 40 minutes, then drink.

WINTER

Beetroot, Carrot and Orange Juice

(*1 serving*)

1 smallish beetroot

4 carrots

1 orange

Juice all ingredients together and drink.

Immunity Broth

(*6 servings*)

1 whole chicken (skin and bones removed)

3 onions, finely chopped

3 carrots, chopped

3 sticks celery, chopped

2 cloves garlic

8cm(2.5inch) piece of ginseng

1 cup mushrooms (shitake or *reishi*)

2 ¾ litres water

Sea salt to taste

Red chilli, finely chopped, to taste

Put all ingredients in a non-metallic pot and slowly bring to the boil. Simmer for about 2 ½ hours. Strain and drink.

Qi for Sounder Sleep

"When a person's body receives something it is real; when the mind receives something it produces dreams."

—Ancient Chinese saying (unattributed)

Sleep is not an optional activity but a biological imperative that does far more than simply rest the body. It heightens the senses, sharpens the mind and mellows the spirit.

Although it is generally accepted that eight hours' sleep each night is optimal, the average woman (aged between 30 and 60 years) sleeps only six hours and forty-one minutes each night during a typical working week. In addition, hormonal fluctuations disrupt sleep patterns for an average of two to three days a month.

In Chinese medicine, the body enters its calm yin phase after midnight, taking over from its active daytime yang *Qi*. Staying up past midnight works against these natural bio-circadian rhythms so to keep in good health we should stay in tune with nature by sleeping during the calming night-time hours. Exercise is best performed early in the morning when yang *Qi* is most active.

To be in top mental and physical form, we need plenty of Rapid Eye Movement or REM sleep in which brainwaves are active and we dream. When a person is *physically* tired it is easier to maintain brainwave activity and sleep generally comes easily. However, someone who is *mentally* exhausted often finds it difficult to sleep (as brainwaves have been overextended). In this case, bedtime stimulants like Walnut and Wolfberry Soup or Cocoa and Wolfberry Smoothie (page 192) help re-energize overworked brain cells, thereby enticing deeper sleeping rhythms.

DREAMING

The active eye motions of REM sleep are believed to occur as the dreamer is actually "watching" their dreams. Ancient Chinese classics related dreams to the wandering of the mind (and/or the soul) and associated various types of unpleasant dreams and nightmares to disharmony within the body (see Dream Interpretations, opposite).

When the body is in harmony, sleep will be deep and few dreams will be remembered. Although difficult to interpret in a rational way (as they rarely make too much sense on waking), dreams are believed by many Chinese medicine practitioners to reveal *Qi* imbalances in the internal organs. For example, dreams connected with water and drowning are symptomatic of a kidney *Qi* deficiency, waking in dream-induced tears is associated with lung disharmony and waking with laughter suggests an imbalance in the heart. With a clearer understanding of how the Five Elements and organs function you can start to interpret your own dreams and become more in tune with your body.

Chinese medicine also recognizes dreams as expressions of unresolved feelings. For example, violence in dreams may be the release of suppressed longing, while the death of a friend or relative in a dream may mean that you are in the process of releasing yourself from an emotional attachment to that person.

Difficulty falling asleep, waking during the night, excessive dreams (leading to restless sleep) and nightmares are extremely common complaints indicative of disrupted *Qi*. The latter can be caused by eating a large meal late in the evening: "If your stomach is uncomfortable, so will be your sleep," dictate the ancient scholars.

Many women (especially those approaching menopause) find they urinate frequently during the night. This is indicative of kidney *Qi* deficiency. If kidney *Qi* is strengthened with foods and herbs, its partner organ (the bladder) will learn to hold urine through the night.

As some of the body's key meridians terminate in the feet, soaking feet in essential oil-infused warm water (about 40°C/105°F) for a minimum of 10 minutes before bed and using gentle reflexology-based massage movements can release tension and induce a more peaceful rest.

DREAM INTERPRETATIONS, CHINESE-STYLE

Crying	Lung excess
White objects or blood	Lung deficiency
Laughter	Heart excess
Fire and smoke	Heart deficiency
Floods and fear	Yin excess
Falling	Fullness in the "lower burner" (pericardium)
Flying	Emptiness in the "lower burner" (pericardium)
Fire	Yang excess
Killing and destruction	Yin and yang excess
Anger	Liver excess
Fright	Gall bladder and heart deficiency
Water and drowning, swimming after a shipwreck	Kidney deficiency
Large cities	Small intestine deficiency
Open fields	Large intestine deficiency
Attack and destruction	Tapeworms in the intestine

TIPS TO INDUCE SOUNDER SLEEP

❖ **Eat earlier and eat less (follow the "75 per cent rule", see page 51)**

❖ **"Relax the heart first and then rest the eyes." Don't bring anger to bed.**

   A calm and still mind induces more peaceful sleeping patterns.

❖ **Exercise in the morning when yang *Qi* is at its peak.**

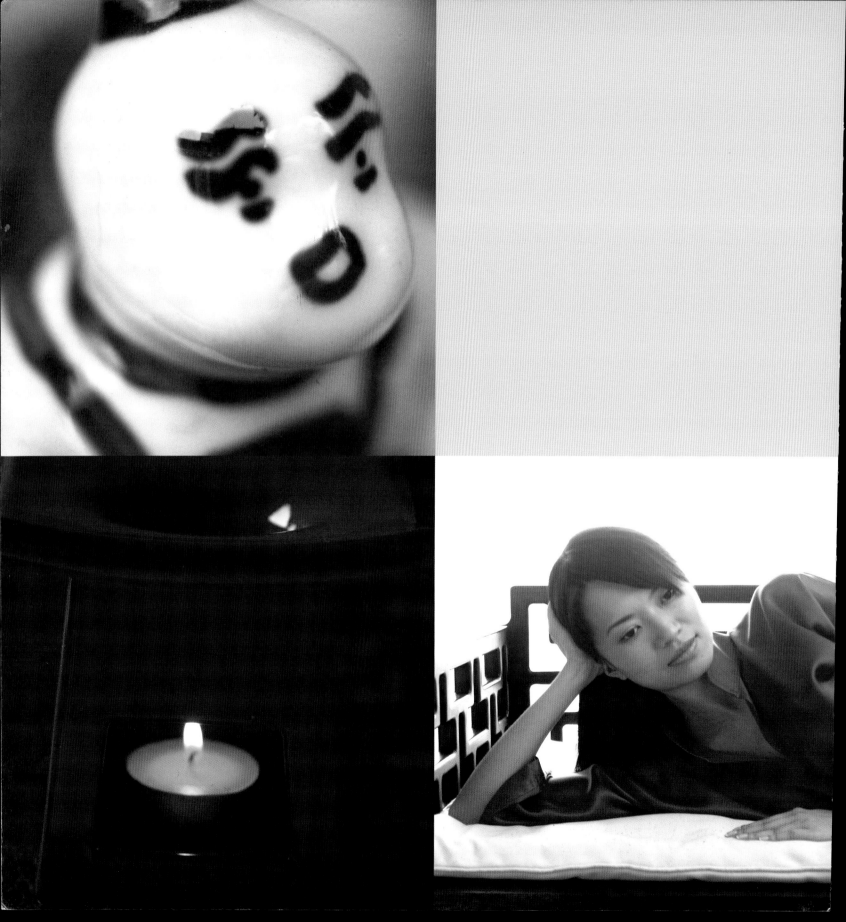

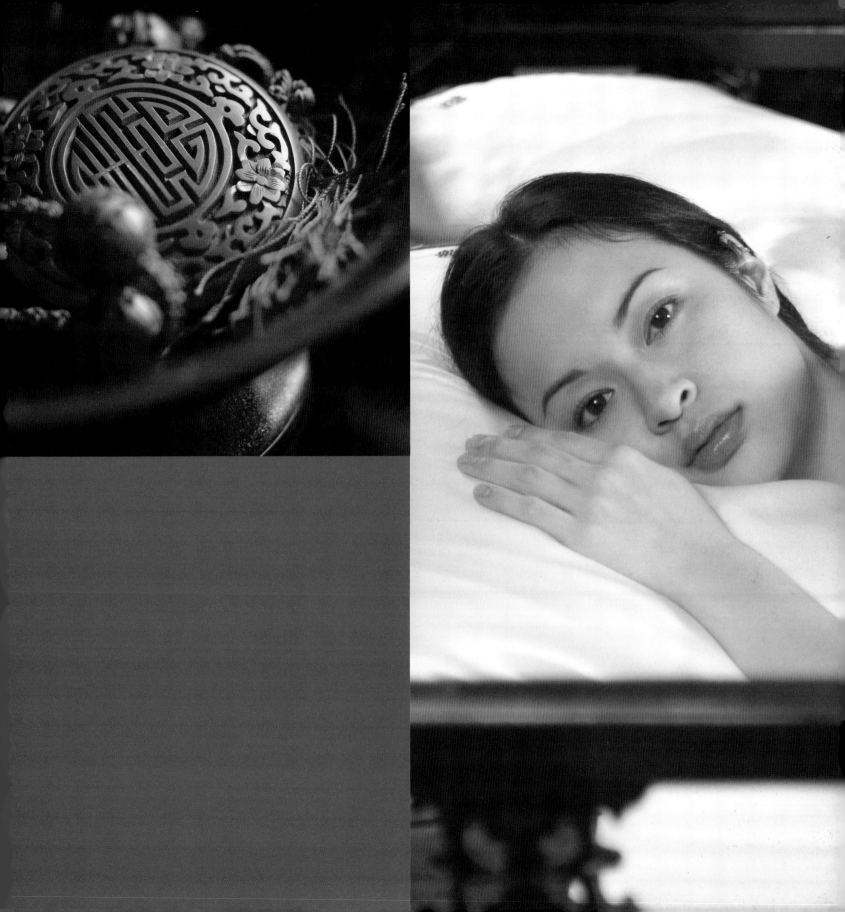

- ⬧ Do not nap during the day.
- ⬧ If physically exhausted or stressed, calming teas like chamomile and peppermint help relax the body and mind. If mentally exhausted, try drinks like Walnut and Wolfberry soup or Cocoa and Wolfberry Smoothie (see page 192).
- ⬧ Let the early morning sunlight fill the bedroom with energy to stimulate wakefulness; keep the curtains open or blinds up through the night.
- ⬧ Burn essential oils of lavender and chamomile in the bedroom before going to bed.
- ⬧ A relaxing massage helps the body physically unwind.
- ⬧ Go to bed and rise at a similar time every day including on weekends.
- ⬧ A gently declining body temperature triggers the onset of sleep so take a bath one hour or so before retiring (and keep bedroom cool).
- ⬧ The bedroom should be as peaceful as possible.
- ⬧ Cut out stimulants like caffeine after 4pm.
- ⬧ Avoid strenuous exercise (other than sex) just before going to bed.

Recommended Chinese herbal formulations:

Emperor's Teapills (Tian Wang Bu Xin Dan) from Plum Flower Brand.

Dosage: Eight tablets three times a day.

Zizyphus Decoction Pills (Suan Zao Ren Tang) from Plum Flower Brand.

Dosage: Two to three tablets, two to three times a day.

Sleep Inducer (Zaoren Anshen Wan) from Tong Ren Tang.

Dosage: 10ml at night before retiring.

Ning Shen Pills from Eu Yan Sang.

Dosage: As recommended by a Chinese medicine practitioner.

QI FLOW CLOCK

Every 24 hours, *Qi* flows continuously through the body in a specific pattern such that for each two-hour period, one organ is dominant. For example, the peak energy for the lungs is between 3am and 5am and someone suffering from a lung complaint or cough may find themselves waking during this time. The kidney ebbs between 5am and 7am when many people wake to urinate.

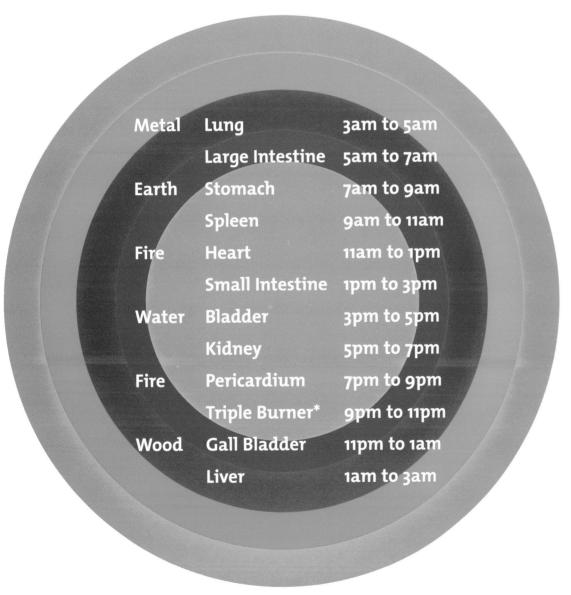

Metal	Lung	3am to 5am
	Large Intestine	5am to 7am
Earth	Stomach	7am to 9am
	Spleen	9am to 11am
Fire	Heart	11am to 1pm
	Small Intestine	1pm to 3pm
Water	Bladder	3pm to 5pm
	Kidney	5pm to 7pm
Fire	Pericardium	7pm to 9pm
	Triple Burner*	9pm to 11pm
Wood	Gall Bladder	11pm to 1am
	Liver	1am to 3am

* Combination of upper, middle and lower burners which in TCM are collectively described as controlling the circulation of bodily fluids.

Recipes for Sounder Sleep

Walnut and Wolfberry Soup

(*2 servings*)

12 skinned walnuts

40g/1.6oz wolfberries

1 1/2 tbsp honey

1 cup water

Blend berries, walnuts and water until the mixture is fine.

Pour into an earthenware pot and bring to the boil.

Remove from heat, add honey, mix, and serve hot.

Cocoa and Wolfberry Smoothie

(*2 servings*)

10g/0.4oz wolfberries

1 tbsp cocoa powder

10g/0.4oz hazelnuts

1 cup soya milk

1 tbsp natural yoghurt

Mix cocoa powder with a tablespoon of warm water before adding to the rest of the ingredients. Blend together and serve.

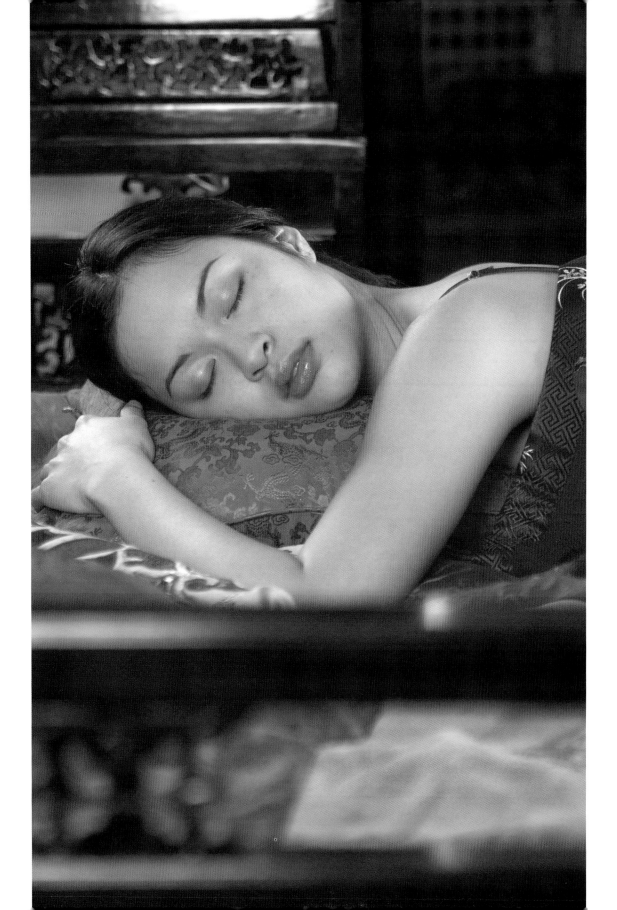

Resources

Banyan Tree Spa Shanghai
Level 3
The Westin Shanghai
Bund Center
88 Henan Central Road
Shanghai, 200002
China
Tel: (86-21) 6335 1888
Fax: (86-21) 6335 2888
rsvns-shanghai@westin.com
www.westin.com/shanghai

Eu Yan Sang International Ltd
269A South Bridge Road
Singapore 058818
Tel: (65) 6225 3211
Fax: (65) 6225 8276
joanna.wong@euyansang.com.sg
www.euyansang.com

Plum Flower Brand
c/- Mayway Corporation
1338 Mandela Parkway
Oakland, California 94607
USA
Tel: (510) 208 3113
Fax: (510) 208 3069
email: info@mayway.com
www.mayway.com

Shanghai Tang
The Pedder Building
Central
Hong Kong
Tel: (852) 2525 7333
Fax: (852) 2530 1888
www.shanghaitang.com

Tong Ren Tang
c/- Chinese Medicine Australian Company
16-20 Sultram Place
Adelaide
South Australia 5000
Australia
Tel: (61-8) 8211 9898
Fax: (61-8) 8231 6799
heidi@chinesemedicineaust.com.au
www.chinesemedicineaust.com.au

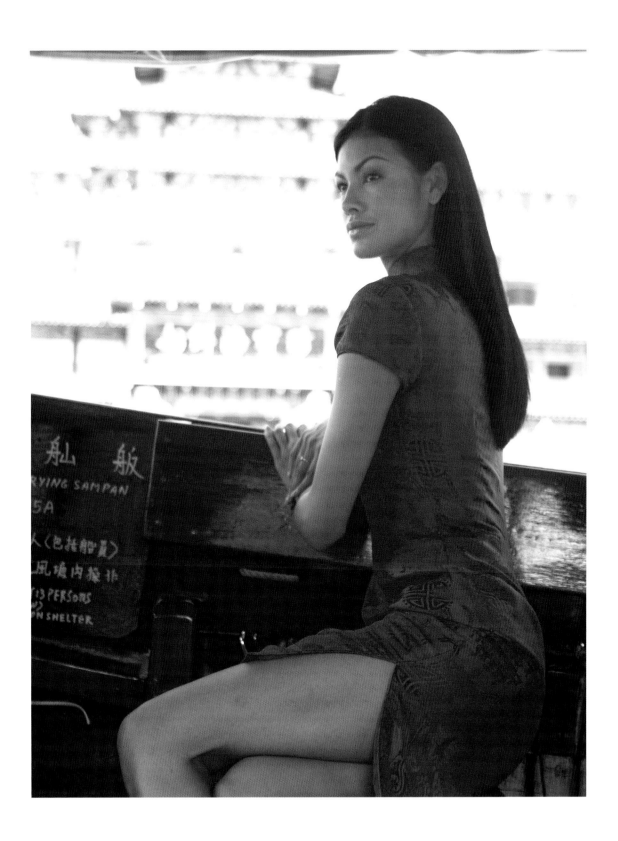

Bibliography

260 Essential Chinese Medicinals, Bob Flaws,
Blue Poppy Press, 1999.

A Dictionary of Chinese Symbols, Wolfram Eberhard,
Routledge, Taylor & Francis Group, 1986.

A Natural Guide to Weight Loss that Lasts, Nan Lu,
HarperCollins Publishers Inc., 2000.

Anti-Ageing Recipes with 100 Chinese Herbs, Tai Li Xiang,
Popular Book Co. Hong Kong, 2000.

Best Selections of Chinese Soup, Zhe Ke Wah, South
Universe, 1999.

Chinese Massage Manual, Sarah Pritchard, Lothian Books,
1999.

Chinese Medical Palmistry: Your health in your hand, Xiao-fan Zong &
Gary Liscum, Blue Poppy Press, 1999.

Chinese Natural Cures: Traditional Methods for Remedies and Treatment,
Henry C Zhu, Black Dog & Leventhqal Publishers, 1994.

Chinese System of Foods for Health & Healing, Henry C. Zhu,
Sterling Publishing Co. Inc., 2000.

Clinical Handbook of Internal Medicine, Vol I,
Jane Lyttleton & Will Maclean, Western Sydney
University Press, 1998.

Guarding the Three Treasures, Daniel Reid, Simon & Schuster,
1993.

Harmony Rules, The Chinese Way of Health Through Food,
Gary Butt & Frena Bloomfield, Samuel Weiser Inc., 1987.

Healthy Recipes with 100 Chinese Herbs, Tai Li Kum,
Popular Book Co. Hong Kong, 2001.

Human Reproduction 11: Reduction of blood flow
impedance in the uterine arteries of infertile women
with electroacupuncture, p1314-1317, E. Stener-Victorin,
U. Waldenstrom, S. Andersson & M. Wilkand, 1996.

Human Reproduction 14: A prospective randomized
study of electroacupuncture versus alfentanil as anaesthesia
during oocyte aspiration in in-vitro fertilization,
p2480-2484, E. Stener-Victorin, U. Waldenstrom,
S. Andersson & M. Wilkand, 1999.

Infertility: Finding the Right Solution, Teoh Eng Soon,
Times Books International, 1987.

Recipes I with Chinese Herbs, Zhe Ke Wah & Qiu Su Zhong,
South Universe, 1999.

Recipes II with Chinese Herbs, Zhe Ke Wah & Qiu Su Zhong,
South Universe, 1999.
Recipes III with Chinese Herbs, Zhe Ke Wah & Qiu Su Zhong,
South Universe, 1999.

Recipes for Pregnancy & Confinement, Patsie Cheong,
Popular Book Co. Hong Kong, 2003.

Staying Healthy with the Seasons, Elson M. Haas, 21st Century
Edition: Celestial Arts, 2003.

The Dancing Wu Li Masters, Gary Zukav, Rider/Hitchinson,
1979.

*The Tao of Beauty: Chinese Herbal Secrets to Feeling Good and Looking
Great,* Helen Lee, Broadway Books, 1999.

The Tao of Healthy Eating, Bob Flaws, Blue Poppy Press, 2002.

The Tao of Health, Sex and Longevity, Daniel Reid, Fireside, 1989.

The Way of Chinese Herbs, Michael Tierra, Pocket Books, 1998.

The Yellow Emperor's Classic of Internal Medicine: Simple Questions
(Huang Ti Nei Jing Su Wen), Original Notes (Tang
Dynasty) Bing Wang, translated by Nelson Liansheng Wu &
Andrew Qi Wu, China Science Technology Press, 2002.

Total Health for Women, Michard & Torg,
Rodale Press Inc., 1995.

Traditional Chinese Medicine: A Natural Guide to Weight Loss that Lasts,
Nan Lu, Quill, 2000.

Women, Hormones & the Menstrual Cycle, Ruth Tricky,
Allen & Unwin, 1998.

Wood becomes Water: Chinese Medicine in Everyday Life, Gail
Reichstein, Kodansha America, Inc, 1998.

Kate O'Brien

Born and educated in Ireland, Kate has a background in nutrition and 15 years' experience in the health, beauty and spa industries in London, Dublin, Singapore and Hong Kong. She is a regular contributor to newspapers and lifestyle magazines in Asia and Australia including *Asia Spa, Harper's Bazaar, Luxury Travel* and the *South China Morning Post.*

Troy Sing, O.M.D.

An Oriental Medical Doctor with extensive training in traditional and modern medicine, Troy runs a successful private practice in Hong Kong. He holds a degree in Chinese Medicine (Acupuncture) from Victoria University in Melbourne, Australia, has completed postgraduate studies at the Beijing College of Traditional Chinese Medicine and spent two years working with Chinese medicine in drug and alcohol rehabilitation programs. Troy holds a Master of Science from the University of Hong Kong. He is an honorary lecturer at the University of Hong Kong's Traditional Chinese Medicine Department and the president of the Hong Kong Medical Acupuncture Association. His research interests include gynaecology and muscular skeletal pain management.

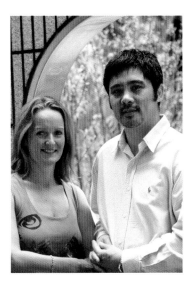

Chester Ong

Born and raised in the Philippines, Chester is currently based in Hong Kong. He specializes in architecture, interiors, food, lifestyle and documentary photography. His work has been featured extensively worldwide.

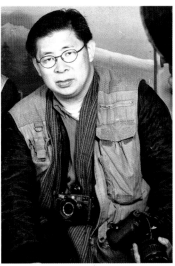

Index

Recipes in bold

Acknowledgements

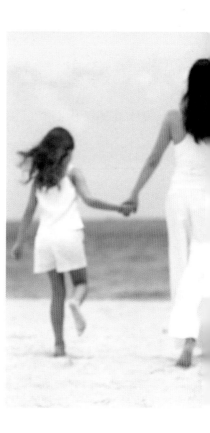

Qi! Chinese Secrets of Health, Beauty & Vitality would not have been possible without ongoing support from family, friends and colleagues. We especially want to thank the following for their enthusiasm throughout the project: Ruth du Cann, our super stylist for her trojan efforts well beyond the call of duty; her product assistant Esther Van Wijck; make-up artists Christine Kohut and Savoy Peng; photographer Chester Ong and his assistants Koon Ming Tan and Michael Lucas; models Rosemary Vandenbroucke, Natalia, Jessie, Leah and Jane; Loretta Reilly, designer extraordinaire in New York; trichology guru Philip Kingsley and his personal assistant Claire Edgecombe in London; Lucy Whittaker, Vicky Neal and Bery Siu of the Paua Group in Hong Kong; Aideen Allan from Aln Design in Dublin and Laura Walsh in Hong Kong for their fabulous graphics and input; Claire Chiang, executive director, Banyan Tree Gallery, and Maisy Koh, corporate director, brand management at Banyan Tree in Singapore (who kindly allowed us to use the symbols on pages 18 and 134, sourced the photographs on pages 9 and 163 and arranged the photo shoot at Banyan Tree Spa Shanghai yielding the images on pages 10, 20, 74, 76, 88, 91, 93, 94, 99, 115, 129, 141, 144, 148, 149, 158, 161, 165, 166, 169 and the back cover); Jariya Tantithakhon and the staff at Banyan Tree Spa Shanghai; Angel Mao at The Westin Shanghai; Sean Harrington, Lisa McCabe and Vicky Bellerby of Elemis in London (responsible for the pictures on pages 74, 95, 96, 98, 103, 138, 142, 155, 169, 182, 183, 198 and 199); Liang Zhong Chen, O.M.D., and Heidi Zschech from the Chinese Medicine Australian Company; Joanna Wong at Eu Yan Sang International in Singapore; Shanghai Tang in Hong Kong for clothes and interiors; TSMK Shanghai and Hong Kong for the use of their restaurant interiors; Dora Tong in Hong Kong for her valuable assistance; and last, but by no means least, Jane Marsden, editor and publisher, Kate's husband Mike and Troy's family for their constant support, enthusiasm and belief in *Qi!*

Yours in health,

KATE O'BRIEN

TROY SING, O.M.D.

May 2005